The Complete Book of Rolfing

The Complete Book of Rolfing

Using the New Physical Therapy To Restructure Your Life

Gary W. Reid

Drake Publishers Inc. New York London

Illustrations by Kip Rosser

Published in 1978 by
Drake Publishers, Inc.
801 Second Avenue
New York, N.Y. 10017

Library of Congress Cataloging in Publication Data

Reid, Gary W.
   The complete book of rolfing.

   Includes index.
   1. Rolfing. I. Title.
RC489.R64R43   615'.822   77-88950
ISBN 0-8473-1669-6

CONTENTS

Acknowledgment

The author wishes to express his thanks to
Mr. Michael L. Case and to Mr. Ken Maryanovich
for their assistance.

*I dedicate this book to the memory of
my grandmother, Mrs. A.E. Goodwin,
my grandfather, Mr. Adam Reid, and
to my brothers and sisters, Bob, Joan,
Jimmy, and Barbara.*

The Complete Book of Rolfing

FOREWORD

I wrote this book out of my deep concern for both the physical and emotional well-being of my fellow man and from my own profound interest in health and mental stability.

If you think highly of yourself and have a certain amount of self-pride, you feel much better physically. People lack initiative and ambition mainly because they don't have the self-confidence to feel that they are capable of accomplishing anything. The people who excel are the ones who discover that they *can* do it. Through venturing forth, they find they are capable of advancing beyond their expected dreams. Such a person is Ida P. Rolf, the founder of rolfing.

Chapter 1

THE HUMAN MACHINE

In modern medicine the discovery of new cures has slowed down, and doctors are taking a look at what they have missed in the past. Human environment and habits, usually taken for granted, are being explored to see if they don't play a part in mental breakdowns, chronic diseases, and poor health in general. There are some patterns which are a forewarning.

As we all know, the body is made up of bones, flesh, and blood. The powerhouse behind the running of this machine is the energy generated by the combination of all the organs, fluid, and systems working together as one. If there is a change, no matter how slight, then a certain amount of interruption takes place, and there is a drainage. This creates a lack of energy, both mentally and physically. Mentally, there is depression or lack of self-confidence. Physically, the body becomes uncomfortable or actually changes in structure. All this is a pattern leading directly to poor health.

In general, the average person is not aware of any of this because all he or she is conscious of is what is visible. This is why we have obesity, people with poor posture, and those who are generally in poor health. They slide into ruts and stay there because they resign themselves to their states due to lack of will power or to the feeling that society does not accept them.

Proper body functioning and good health go together as one. Without good health the body won't function properly, and without proper body functioning, it is impossible to have good health. The body won't tire as easily when the mind is not as tormented and in a healthier and more relaxed state.

People tend to take too many things for granted. This includes their physical health. Only in the past five to ten years has the interest in physical exercise that existed back in the postwar days returned on a daily basis. This includes bicycling, jogging, swimming, and skiing. The whole point is that people are becoming more and more health conscious. The problem is that they have let it go a little too long, and after so many years, their bodies have become limp objects of flabby flesh and sagging bone. In order to return to a state of good health, the framework must be in proper structural form.

If we take a good look around us, at our families and friends, we see a lack of balance and limb coordination. As an instructor in physical education for over ten years, I have had to deal with this problem from the start. People are not symmetrically aligned; when the spine is out of alignment, it affects the neck and the position of the head. In our society today, people overeat, and a heavy body, supported by small legs, gives a force of great downward pressure. The belly is too large in comparison to the chest. This throws the whole balance out of whack, and nothing creates a solid structure. It takes no trained medical eye to spot these problems in average people on the street. The overall body may well be four to six inches out of position.

The following illustrations show a few of the abnormal physical positions common in most people when sitting, standing, sleeping, bending, and lifting a package. See if you recognize a few of your friends, or even yourself, in these pictures (Figs. 1-1, 1-2, 1-3, 1-4, and 1-5).

These people exist in all strata of society. They may state that they are in good shape, but in reality they are not very happy with their physical structures. They hide their anxieties in a shroud of excuses. These excuses range anywhere from popping pep pills or downers to seeking professional help. Doctors are continuously hampered by the psychological problems of patients. If these people felt better about themselves emotionally, they would find out they are not really physically ill.

Someone who is sick feels either that medicine will cure it, or else it has to be an injury. It takes a very strong-willed person to admit the need for psychiatric help. There are too many excuses as to why we do not feel well or do not function properly. Whether it is grief, anger, anxiety, or another mood, it all stems from within.

*The average person
is not aware of a change
in physical structure
that may lead to poor health.
Bad posture while standing or sitting
causes a lack of energy,
both physically and mentally.*

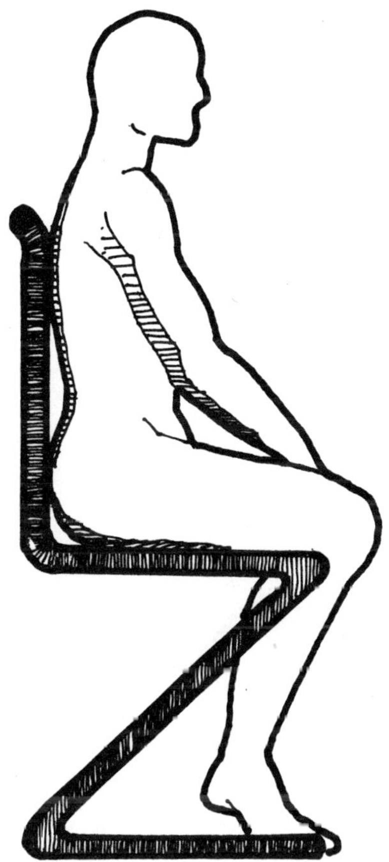

Figure 1-1

SITTING

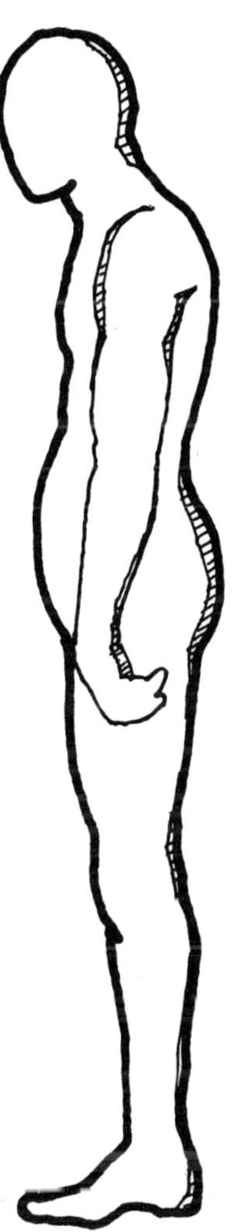

Figure 1-2

STANDING

If we take a look around us,

we see a lack of balance and limb coordination

in our families and friends.

Being the right weight for your height

doesn't necessarily mean

that you are healthy.

Proper physical alignment is essential.

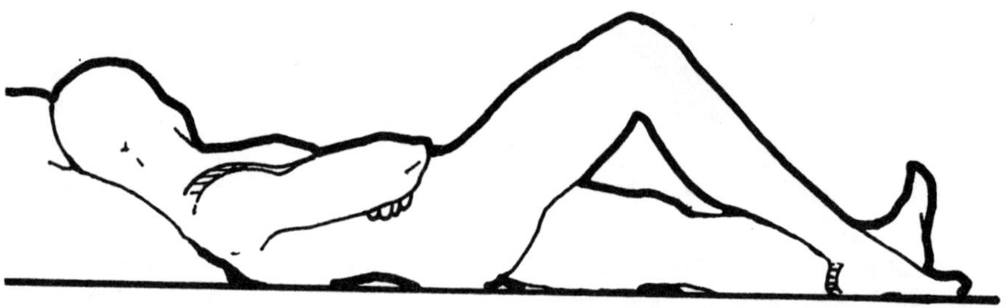

Figure 1-3

SLEEPING

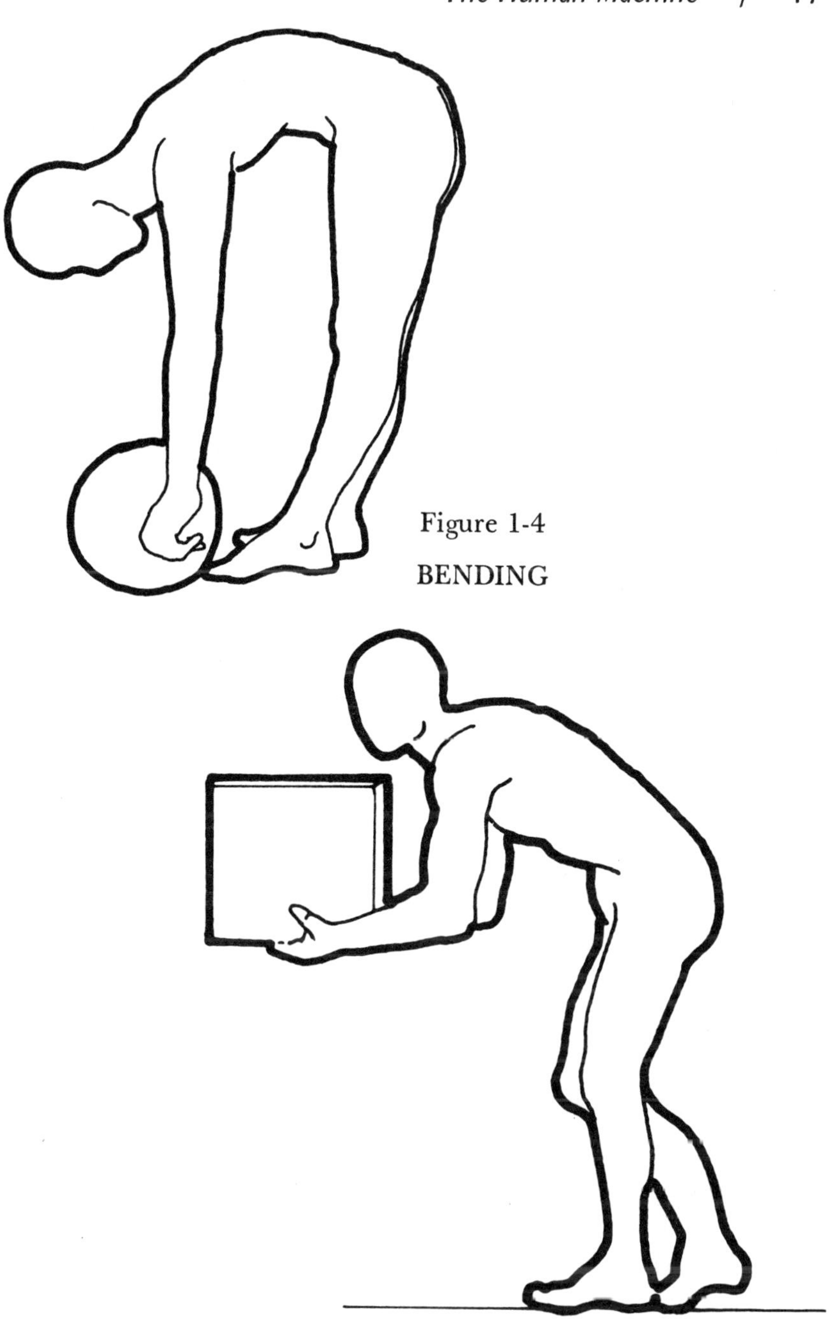

Figure 1-4

BENDING

Figure 1-5

LIFTING A PACKAGE

To many people there seems to be no cure for what is wrong with them. The closest the West has come to soul-searching is psychoanalysis. I really feel that man is searching too far and looking for too much of a problem when the possible answer lies in how he feels about himself. Psychology is okay to remedy some emotional problems, but what about feeling down, depressed, and moody to the point that the body chemistry becomes upset and changes, causing a personality change. These changes can be caused not only by unbalanced diets, but how about physical structure. If the machine is not functioning properly, then the running and the production of the machine must be affected.

There is a new approach to human malfunctions, both physical and psychological. We run, much too often, to our doctors to look for a cure. This is usually in the form of therapy or medicine. If people simply looked after their own personal machines better and kept them in better condition, there would be no problems.

Simply looking good or being the right weight for your height doesn't always mean that you are healthy. The body must be functioning right inside in order to be in good shape — healthy. We believe if we look healthy and we don't hurt physically, then we are all right. This is definitely wrong. It's like trying to guess a person's occupation by his dress.

From early youth to well into our adult lives, we continuously abuse ourselves physically without really knowing it. Remember, if we don't hurt, then we figure we are all right. The same goes for our minds. Our minds are conditioned to certain patterns from childhood on and play a most important part in the forming of our personalities. If the body or mind is abused in youth, it will act up later in life. These damages may result from a simple twist of the body, a slight bump, or from merely standing, sitting, or sleeping improperly.

A child will simply assume that other children are better at certain things than he is and will compensate for it in another way, either physically or psychologically. The parent will almost never realize the cause of the emotional strain on the child due to this fact. The parent will feel that there is something wrong physically and take the child to a medical doctor who will describe the child as healthy. This simple unbalance is extremely difficult to notice, whether by a layman or by a trained professional. Doctors in the East have managed to recognize this and deal with the patient both emotionally and physically. It is called a harmonious balance within a person. It is only recently that the West has begun to realize the patient must be treated as a whole.

Genetics is another factor. A problem, be it psychological or physical, may be inherited.

Our bodies are vast systems of bone structure and tissue, run by a myriad of tubes and organs which take care of the chemistry in order to give us energy to run on. Any slight deviation in this system will cause some failure or damage. It seems strange to have something wrong and then find out that it started twenty years previously.

This whole discussion on the running of the human machine leads up to a form of treatment, not yet heard of by everyone, called "rolfing." Basically rolfing means the structuring of the body into alignment. This book is written in order to give the layman a knowledge of the why, where, and how of rolfing.

Chapter 2

SUPPORTIVE PRINCIPLE

The human form is structured so that every part has its proper place, and each piece interlocks with each other in order for the body to function properly. It is like piling things up so that they won't fall over or constructing a building. If each piece is not in its proper place, then the structure will falter or fall.

As we know, everything is pulled downward by gravity. Therefore, if everything is not set in its proper place, it will be pulled out and down causing a misalignment in the body. What actually should be done is the same as grabbing someone by the hair and lifting him straight up until he is fully stretched and hanging in a perfectly vertical position. This may be easily fixed in youth, but in adulthood, it becomes more complicated. Simply putting one piece back in its proper position does not alter the situation. All pieces must be properly placed in order to have a perfect alignment, and then the human bag of skin may work right. This creates a strain-free system. The illustration shows the result of poor physical structure (Fig. 2-1).

The top half of the body has a heavier concentration of weight which increases with the added weight of the pelvic region and the lower extremities. This weight buildup is the same as the concentrated weight of a 145-pound woman in high heels. As the cumulative weight builds up on its way to the high heel of the shoe, so does the amount of pressure per square inch on every part of the body. By the time the pressure hits the heel, there is a concentrated force of about 1,500-2,000 pounds per square inch on the one spot. This sounds a little unbelievable, but it is true.

With all the running, walking, sitting, and standing we do, along with the twisting and straining, it is no wonder that the pulling of these parts by the tendons and muscles dislodges the joints and

Every part of the body must be properly placed in order to have a perfect alignment. Otherwise the resulting damage becomes harder to correct.

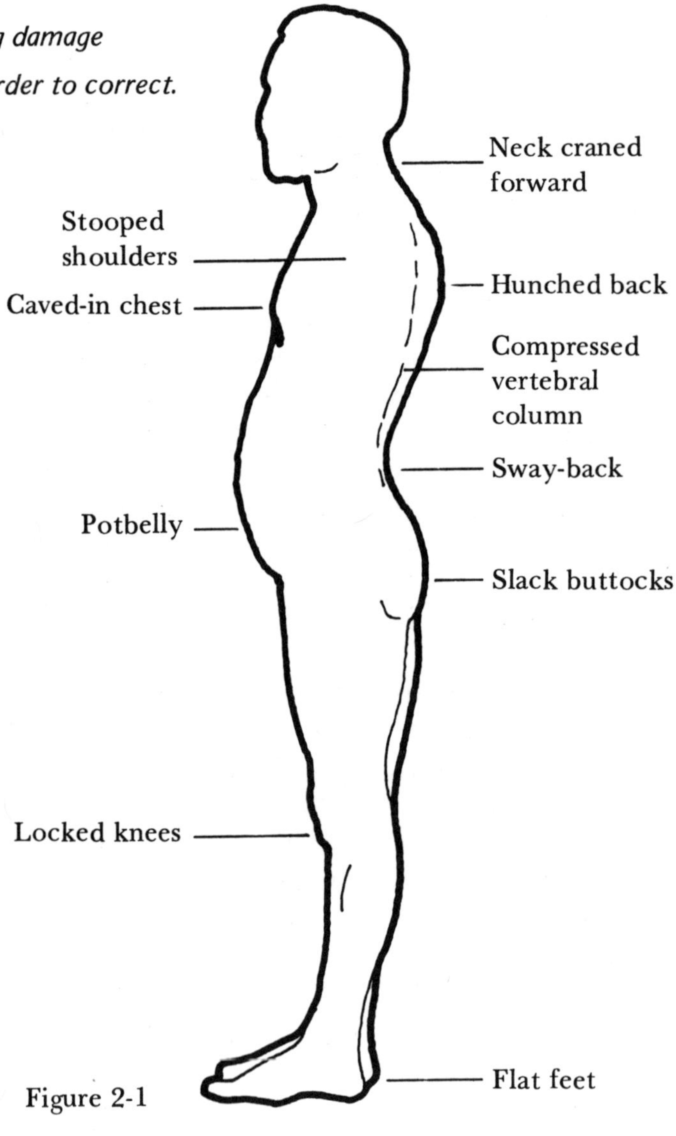

Figure 2-1

blocks the flow of the body chemistries that make the body function properly. Thus, when we reach adult stage, we have done more damage to our bodies and systems than we realize.

Why are people never satisfied with their figures? They always seem to be complaining even when they look like they are in good shape. If asked, they will say they just don't seem to feel right. This "not feeling right" is the sign which means that there is something wrong *inside.* Even after a medical checkup they still feel uncomfortable. That is because the system inside is just not running right, and it is causing an imbalance that can cause aches or pains. Immediately after being rolfed, a patient will state that he simply feels a lot better even though he really doesn't know how or why. The body responds better when the bones, skin, and muscles are in order, each performing its proper function.

Rolfing is not a medical discipline, but a different idea as to what can be wrong when no medical reason may be found. It makes sense when there is no other reason.

STARTING AT THE BOTTOM

As with any structure, you must begin at the bottom in order to cement a solid base for support. Therefore, the feet are the base of the human structure. The feet support the whole weight of the body and help balance it. The feet tell the whole tale as to what is happening above. The next time you are in a public place where people have no shoes on — beaches or public swimming pools — look first at someone's feet and then continue up to the upper part of the body. You will be surprised as to the impression you get. Observing the feet first and following up allows you to see how the rest of the structure is put together and where the pulls and strains exist. Each of these complements the other. The feet reveal the structure, and the structure controls the feet. Observe the illustrations (Fig. 2-2).

Notice how some feet are flatter than others. Some feet turn

*The feet support the weight of the body
and show where
the stresses and strains exist.*

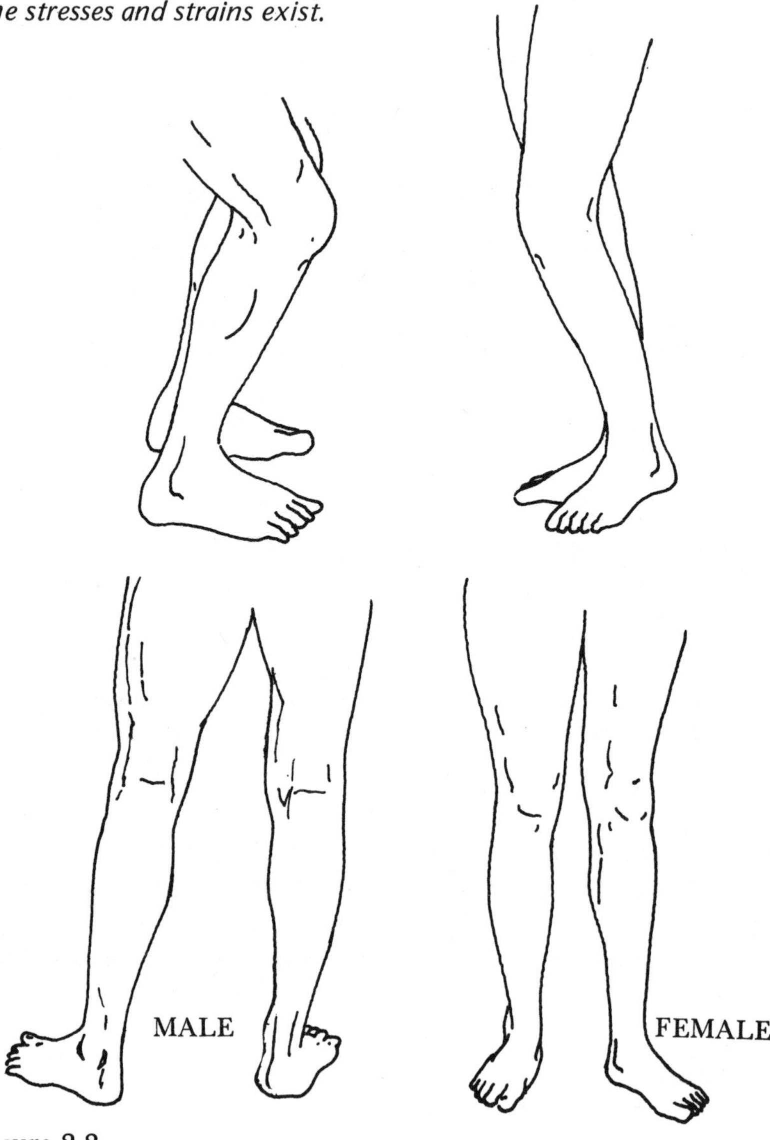

Figure 2-2

in while others turn out. The weight of the body is seen in the feet, and a mental picture of the person can be drawn just by observing the feet. These are the first telltale signs of the problems that exist in the body. If they are out of alignment, then whenever we walk, we pull, twist, and strain the rest of the body. All this leads to structural damage. Aches and pains get worse, and the person involved becomes more mentally distressed or tires more easily when performing everyday functions.

The foot, consisting of twenty-six bones, is constructed to support the weight of the mass above, provided the weight is in proportion to the height (Fig. 2-3). If that weight is too much, it will create a weakness in the supporting foot area. This throws the whole system out of whack. The foot with its arch (Fig. 2-4) is designed to withstand the weight if the individual walks properly, placing the heel down first and following through with the rest of the foot. This way, the weight is distributed evenly over the entire area.

The structure is held together by a series of tendons, muscles, and joints coming together to do their part in the working of the foot, and any interruption in this complex system causes an effect on the whole area, creating a problem not only in the foot, but in the ankle and all the way up to the rest of the body, hampering the way it performs its daily functions. The ankle acts as a hinge or joint and must work like a well-greased machine in order that the weight may be evenly distributed over the foot. The stretchability and the length of the tendons in the working ankle play an important part in the way the weight is distributed over the foot.

If there is a damaged area or a shortening of one of the controlling tendons, then there is an overall effect on performance. The individual will naturally compensate for the problem by forc ing the other parts of the foot to work harder and longer to do the work of the damaged area. This compensation goes on further, all the way up the body. It invariably throws the balance off and makes the feet work harder in the job of supporting the body weight. Adding to all of this, the sole of the foot then has

*The foot consists of twenty-six bones
and helps to balance the body,
as well as to support it.
If the weight is not in proportion
to the height, a weakness
in the supporting area is the result.*

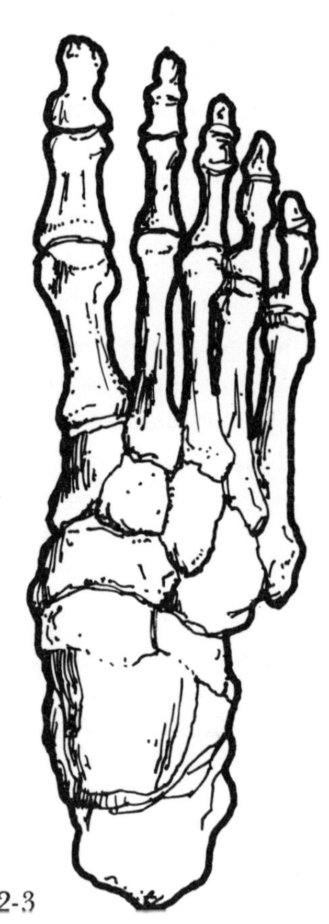

Figure 2-3

The arch of the foot withstands the body's weight
provided the individual walks properly.
The heel comes down first,
followed by the rest of the foot.
The weight should be distributed evenly
over the entire area.

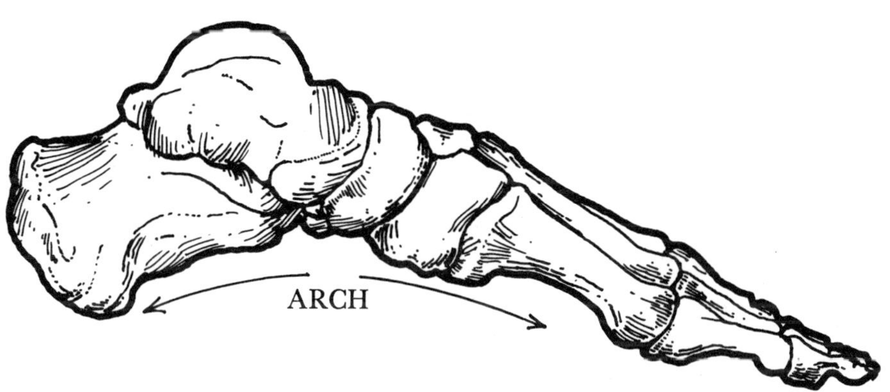

Figure 2-4

to make good contact with the ground, and if there is a malfunction, then it, too, affects the contact and causes adjustments that have to be made in the functioning of the foot. The longer this condition exists, the greater the effect it will have on the overall working of the body (Fig. 2-5).

The leg, from the calf down, contains the stronger muscles which play an important part in the working of the foot. The strength of the muscles in the calf travels to the ankle along tendons, and the ankle becomes a pulley that joins the force of the leg to the foot to give the power to walk. If any part of this system deteriorates, then the section that is included in its functional purpose is also affected, causing a problem in the leg. Notice that an obese person can walk only a short distance before tiring. An observation of footprints immediately shows the differences in the balanced and unbalanced prints.

THE KNEES

The knees are simply joints. As with the ankle, they must be aligned so that the weight is evenly projected coming down on top of the knee so that it can continue on down to the ankle and the foot. Each part must be placed properly on top of the other in order to distribute the weight down to its proper part. If the whole leg is not in functioning order, then the human body has the ability to adjust to a certain degree, even though this adjustment is not always good. This is simply the start of the process of throwing the rest of the body into an adjustment that changes and affects the whole being (Fig. 2-6).

When the knee joints are not functioning properly, the thighs come together, and this tends to force the feet to point outward. When this happens, the tendons and muscles on the outer part of the legs are not stretched and worked as hard as the inner parts, and, therefore, they restrict movement and tend to tighten. Before long, the discomfort disappears, and the walker's gait becomes natural to the point where he is not aware of it. Remember, a child is taught how to stand and walk, and if the child is

*The sole of the foot has to make good contact
with the ground, or other parts of the foot
have to work harder to support the body weight.
Invariably, balance is affected.*

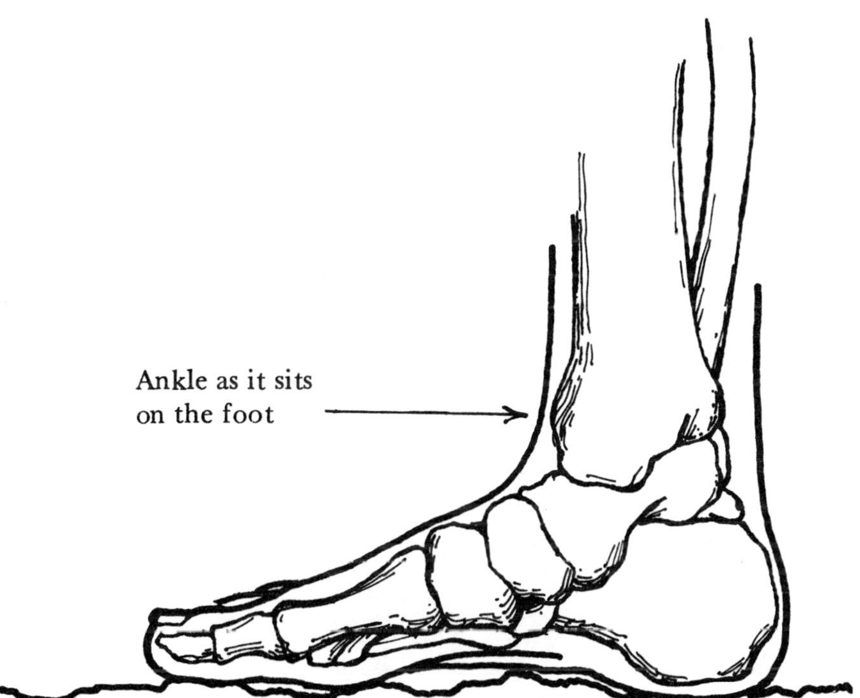

Figure 2-5   FOOT ADJUSTING TO THE CONTOURS
OF THE GROUND

The weight coming down
on top of the knee
must be evenly projected so that
it can continue down to the ankle and foot.
When the knee joint is not functioning
properly, restricted movement results.

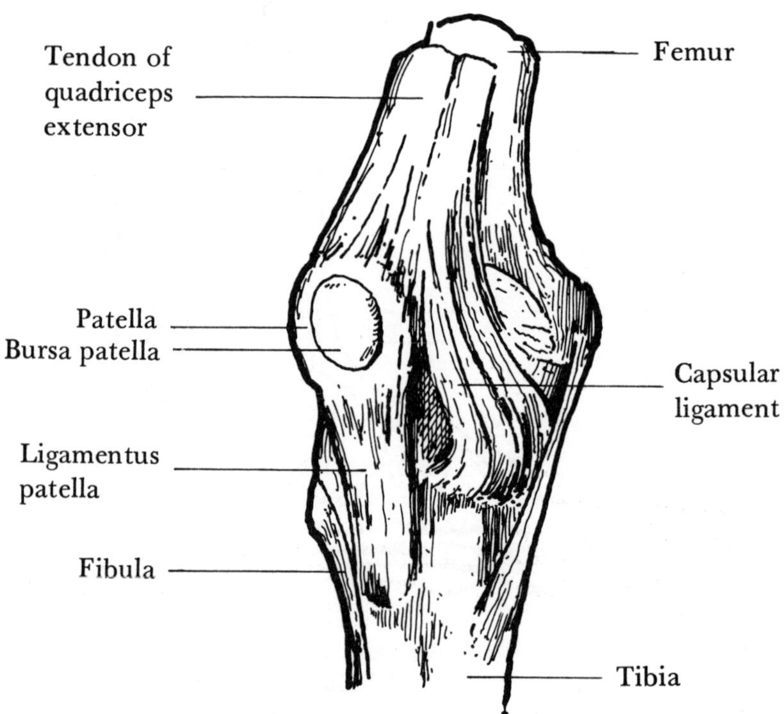

Figure 2-6 . ANTERIOR VIEW OF THE RIGHT KNEE JOINT

taught wrong, he will be unaware of which habits are causing the problems.

Too many people have excuses for physical problems. They say "I was born this way." As Ida P. Rolf states in her book, "Most people are born with unformed skeletal structures, but as they grow, corrections take place naturally to become a proper structure."

Following up the human torso, we can see different gaits from behind. The size of the fatty tissue in the rear plays an indifferent role in the actual problem. In reality, the problem stems from the pelvic bone structure. From the waist, to the knees, and on down to the ankles and feet is the route of the rolfer. The actual walk and the foot imprints are the telltale signs. If the muscle tissue and tendons in the leg cease working or even slow down, then there is a deterioration in their usefulness. When this happens, there is a noticeable problem after a period of time. This occurs in many disabilities and treatments. Take dieting, for instance. The results of dieting can be seen only over a long period of time. The same with the destruction and also the correction of the human body.

The route may be traced up the leg when there is a problem which affects the foot. It will show in the ankle, possibly the knee, and most of the time, in the pelvic area. It may be caused by an accident, a birth defect, or it may come over a long period of time from a simple imbalance caused by a shortened ligament or a misplaced joint. In the latter, the deformation comes only after a long time, and to correct it also takes time. People, whether they are dieting to lose weight, trying to gain weight, or having a nutritional problem corrected, always expect immediate results. When the ankle or hip is damaged, it doesn't always affect the other parts, but when there is damage in the knee area, it affects both the pelvic area and the feet. When the knee is knocked out of whack or even permanently damaged, it changes the structural pattern of the pelvic area which, in turn, reacts on the ability to walk properly.

THE PELVIC REGION

This area has been the central and most important physical part since the beginning of time. It not only supports the whole top half of the human frame, it is the central point of balance. It is also the control center for receiving the messages so that the lower half may function. Depending on the shape and the condition of the body, the pelvis may have a difficult or easy job. If the top half is heavy, then the pelvis must work extra hard to maintain balance. If it must work hard, then the pressure downward will dislodge other sections in the waist, knees, and ankles, causing problems.

The male and female pelves function basically the same way in that they are both the center of balance (Figs. 2-7 and 2-8). When the top half is overly heavy, it creates a shifting in the weight on the bone structure, causing a shift all the way down the line. This, in turn, creates a forward pulling motion on the spine and rib cage that leads to further problems.

Pains such as those of arthritis or rheumatism are caused mostly by a change of body chemistry or by the deterioration of the muscles, tendons, ligaments, and fluids in the system. Some medical experts are far too quick to diagnose pains in the legs and shoulders as arthritis or rheumatism. Through rolfing, the rearranging of the bone structure, most of the aches and pains may be eliminated. Mind you, this is not to say that they can all be fixed by it. The standing position automatically shows the problem to the naked eye (Fig. 2-9).

If the eye follows the form up from the feet, a distinct turn may be seen almost immediately, traveling up from the ankles. This, in turn, affects the waist and the pelvic region that is so important. Notice the side effects in the morning when you rise. You will feel twice as tired and ache when you should feel great and rested after a good night's sleep. You either chalk it up to a rough night before, or say that you are feeling your age. This is, naturally, incorrect.

The pelvic area is the central point of balance
and supports the top half of the human frame.
It is a massive bony ring.
Too much weight above
causes too much pressure on the pelvic bones.

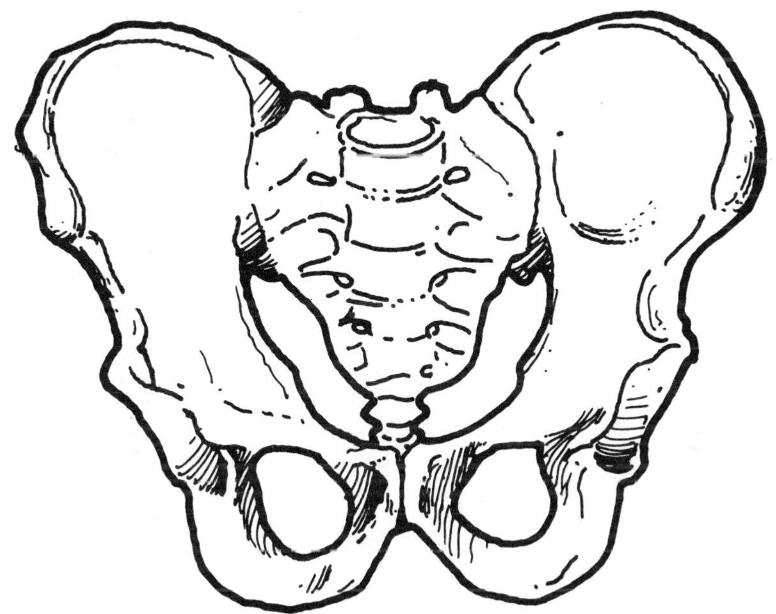

Figure 2-7   ANTERIOR VIEW (MALE)

Both the male and female pelves function basically
the same way as far as balance.
The pelvis rests on the lower extremities
and supports the spine.
Exercise plays an important role
in strengthening the pelvic area,
but it should not be done on a hard surface.

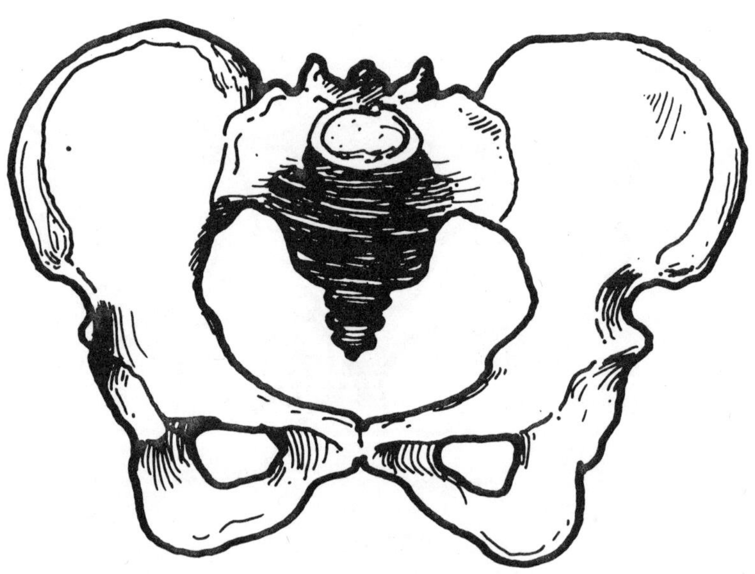

Figure 2-8   ANTERIOR VIEW (FEMALE)

The results of strain
may be followed
from the bottom up.
The feet and ankles
are turned out, and the knees,
pelvis, and waist are pulling.
The body aches and is tired
even after a good night's sleep.

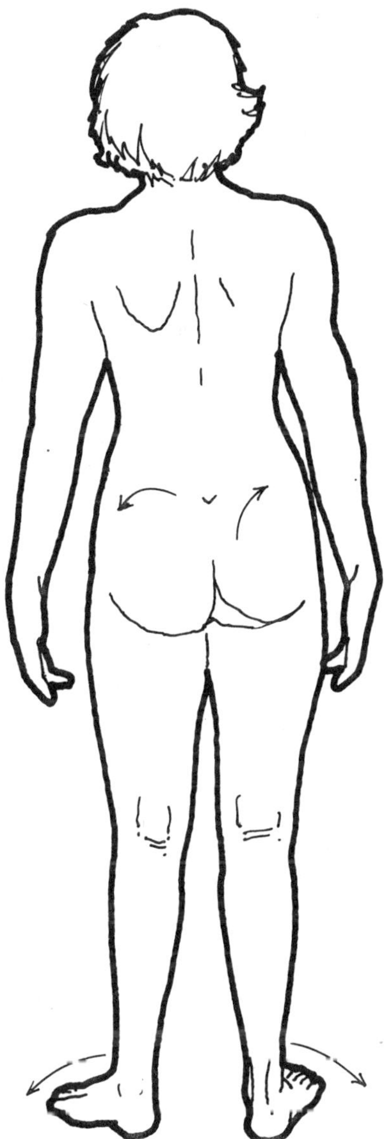

Figure 2-9

Continuing exercise will tighten the muscles and cords of the body even more, and they then cease to function properly. When this happens, the bone structure is restricted in movement, and the frame is thrown off. In a chain reaction, it will affect the whole body. Because these cords and muscles cross the knee and hip joints, the whole body is pulled tighter together, restricting movement, and dislodging other parts, causing them to turn either inward or outward. This, in turn, throws off the whole balance. The first result is that the individual feels slow, tight, and sluggish, and it is easily visible. Flabby men have much the same problem as athletes. Both ways present problems.

Heavy weight above the body causes imbalance and creates "knock-knees" or "pigeon-toes." The chest protrudes, and a totally uncomfortable feeling exists.

The pelvis is merely a joint connecting the upper and lower halves of the body. The base of the foot controls the working of the pelvis by transmitting the structural alignment up the leg. When the pelvis is restricted in movement, it can cause a counter movement in the legs and throw everything out of position. The hip joint must rotate freely so that it will not add to any restrictions. The abdominal or inner controlling tissue must be flexible and strong so that it won't tighten and withhold movement of the ball and joint sockets in the upper legs. Most of the muscles, tendons, and cords generally play an important part in transmitting fluids and foods to different parts of the body. This is also affected by any of the previously mentioned problems. Exercise plays an important role in strengthening the pelvic area. Each exercise has its own part and will serve its purpose if it is not overdone. Exercising is also wrong when it is done on a hard surface.

The *rectus abdominis* muscle begins at the rib cage, and if there is a tightening of the muscles in the area, it will exert a frontal pulling force on the whole upper structure, causing the top half of the body to pull forward from the neck down with the head and neck craned forward. Should this condition continue, it could lead to an unwanted hump in the back.

Rolfing treatment consists of the proper, gradual forcing of each part which, in turn, releases pressure on the muscles and cords and allows the interlocking joints to return to their proper places, correcting the disorders as each joint is fixed.

The *psoas* muscle is one of the most important muscles in the body. It is divided into two sections, the psoas major and the psoas minor. The correct position for this muscle is inverted toward the back of the body. If it becomes straightened rather than inverted from the top of the pelvis down, it causes an "S"-shaped posture with an extended lower abdomen (Fig. 2-10). If this condition exists, it almost always is accompanied by a bad lower back — an arc at the base of the spine and backache.

Beginning at the fifth vertebra and extending downward to the top of the femur at the hip joint, the psoas muscle makes the difference in correct posture. It acts as a steel-like cable joining the upper and lower halves of the body. If the psoas is not responding correctly, then the digestive system is disturbed and constipation is the result. The lumbar nervous system is affected, and this area is completely thrown out of balance. The rib cage becomes sloped downward and forward. Truly erect stance is impossible in this condition. A quick jerk or turn can cause loss of balance. Walking is affected, as well as standing. The psoas must be operating smoothly for effortless walking or standing.

When everything is working properly, the upper part of the torso can sit in a snug comfortable spot with all parts supported evenly. The proper procedure for checking your psoas muscle for any problems is simply to lie on the floor, and, arcing the base of your back, check to see if your stomach protrudes or whether it simply rises up with the rest of the upper torso. Your back should be touching the floor at about the second vertebra up from the base of the spine.

If your stomach protrudes, it could be a definite sign of psoas trouble. Standing, walking, or any movement in an upright position is done in conjunction with the psoas muscle. Anyone — athlete, office worker, or artist — will move with both grace and ease if his body is integrated into one complete unit. In the average person, the psoas muscle is usually sluggish in its working hab-

One of the most important muscles in the body,
the psoas is divided into two sections.
Its correct position is inverted toward
the back of the body. Otherwise, it causes
an "S"-shaped posture
with an extended lower abdomen,
almost always accompanied by a bad lower back.

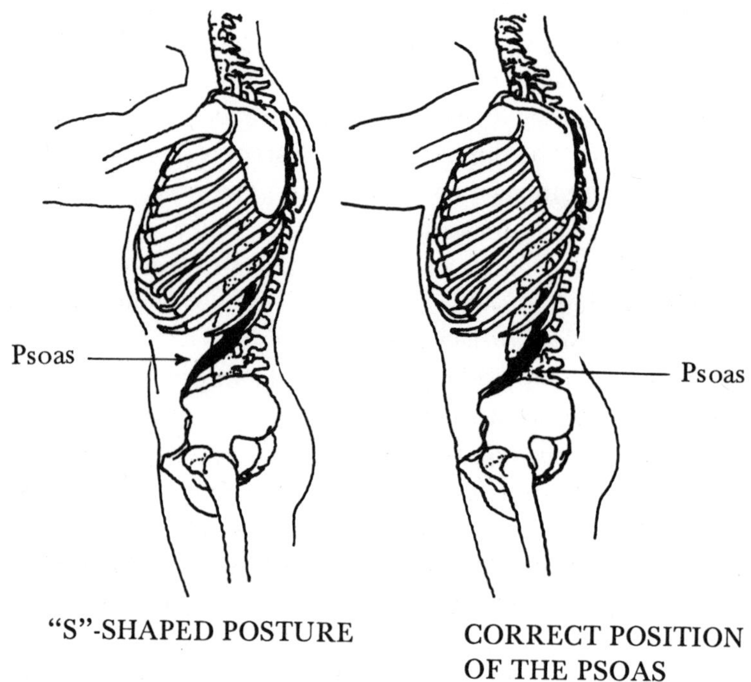

"S"-SHAPED POSTURE   CORRECT POSITION
OF THE PSOAS

Figure 2-10

its and lies flush along the pelvic brim. This almost always means
that the individual is restricting himself to outer physical movement. This lack of use of the psoas muscle will hamper it and
cause it to restrict back on the rectus, leading to future problems.

All movement of the legs originates from the trunk or waist.
The message is transmitted through the psoas muscle, and the
legs follow the order. When the psoas is pulled down tight against
the pelvic brim, the femur or the top of the leg joint must pull
itself around the psoas muscle, which usually results in a side-to-
side gait. The legs should have the ability to move in a straight
forward and backward motion without affecting any other part
of the body.

Another result of a bad psoas is having to pick up your legs
with every movement in walking. When you have to do this, it
causes the stomach muscles to tighten. The continuous effort
involved will cause the wall of the stomach to become either
pouchy or overly tight. The work involved in walking in this
manner will also cause the thigh muscles to tighten to the point
of being trapped in their own mass. This is obvious in weight
lifters, athletes, and dancers. They pay the price with the pains
that accompany this condition when they retire from their pro-
fessions. If the psoas had been functioning properly throughout
their careers, then they would not have to retire as early in life
as they usually do.

The pelvic area, basically a bony mass, supports the structure.
It is held together by the outer layers of skin, bone, and ligaments. One must complement the other in order to function properly. The pelvis and sacrum are, in reality, the base for the spine
to sit upon and are usually viewed as one by the eye of the layman. Actually they are separate and come together to work in
the mature adult. When the psoas stops working properly and
sticks to the pelvic brim, this serves to pull the pelvis outward and,
in turn, affects the spine above and the legs below. Most of the
strain is usually felt around the fourth vertebra and is commonly
referred to as a bad backache. If the psoas is exercised and
worked back into functional order, then the pressure is lessened

in all parts, and the pains go away. Thus, it leads to better posture and working order for the entire back and pelvis.

The *hamstring* muscles and the *gluteus maximus* are the strongest and most powerful muscles in the body. They serve to join the lower part of the leg with the pelvic structure.

The gluteus maximus is the most prominent muscle lying at the back of the hip joint and forms the buttocks. When you run, or climb stairs, it is the main muscle used.

The hamstring muscles originate in the pelvis, extend down the back of the thigh, behind the knee, and into the lower leg bones. They enable you to flex your knees.

These two sets of muscles play an important part in balance, and anytime you see squatty, tight thighs, they are the result of shortened and massy hamstrings. When this happens, restricted movement and poor balance are the result. It is very common for a heavy man to have very weak knee joints. The legs become tight and painful when there is motion. Some of the signs of hamstring muscles in trouble are: a shortening of the neck cords, wider hips, the inability to pull the knees into the chest when lying on your back, and a noticeable imbalance in movement when walking or even standing still. The shortening of the hamstrings tends to pull the knee joint together and can cause twisting in the knee joint itself. A simple example is being unable to come even near touching your toes while standing erect and bending at the waist.

The gluteus muscle may cause many problems if it tightens too much. It forces the femur at the top of the leg to work hard and throws the whole leg itself out. Therefore, its shape and design are very important. As I said earlier, when each part is not functioning properly, then it causes a reaction in another part, and this, in turn, reacts on still another section. It goes back to the theory that the site of the actual problem is not always at the point at which it appears.

In rolfing, the gluteus is massaged and worked continuously, relieving the tension and pressure which allows the muscle to start working like a well-greased cable again. This begins to get all the parts that have been affected back into perspective and working properly again. The heavy hips start to perform more work and thus lose their excess weight and become more compact.

When the *sacrum* cannot move easily and the fatty tissue protecting it becomes stringy, the bony sacrum feels like it is directly next to the skin and can be painful, especially in a person with broad hips. The sacrum's upper point then tends to lean forward, and this is sometimes compensated for by rotation backwards on its apex. The strong ligaments holding the sacrum in place are supposed to prevent this movement. These ligaments that control the movement or the non-movement of the sacrum are really the key to all disorders in the area. They, in turn, are the point of attachment for the leg muscles and the ligaments and cords which control the movement and balance of the lower part of the human structure. A great many people have the problem of forward sacrum tilting.

Muscles and bones interlock in their roles, although in the past, it was thought that they were separately functioning units. For instance, there are three important muscle groups on the floor of the pelvis which allow us to move the pelvic bones as separate units. If there are any problems with these muscles, bladder control is affected. In women, they are very important in childbirth. Women should start a set of exercises immediately after childbirth in order to tone and strengthen these muscles.

Both in the male and the female, sexual orgasm is directly related to the controlled responses of these lower pelvic muscles. If these muscles are not working properly without any restrictions, sexual gratification may be harder to obtain, and frigidity may result due to the lack of the ability to respond. Any inflammation in the area will result in great pain or discomfort during sexual intercourse.

The positioning of the bones and their ability to perform their proper functions rely almost entirely on the proper working of the muscles. The coccyx (the small bones at the base of the sac-

rum) is where these pelvic muscles come together. The coccyx
is joined to the sacrum by only a thin disc and is continuously bat-
tered in everyday life by bumping and sitting down hard. Any
type of knock or fall may cause the coccyx to shift, and when
this happens, the main pelvic muscles are moved, and the whole
pelvic structure is affected. This causes the pelvis to tip, and the
upper and lower parts of the body structure then become affected.
It is seen mainly in the upper half where the stomach is forced forward, and the back area at the base of the neck hunches outward
in a curving arc. Exercise will only cause the muscles and cords
to tighten further and add to the problem. The pelvic and abdominal organs are affected and begin to deteriorate. In the female,
the uterus and the ovaries are lacking support. In the male, the
prostate gland lacks support. The intestinal tract and the bladder
also become affected. Discomfort and depression result.

THE SPINE

The spine acts as a supporting pole which keeps the body upright
and holds it in a straight line from the toes to the top of the head.
It also encases the main line in the body's nervous system. The
central generating units are housed in the base of the spine and in
the base of the skull at the top of the spine. A severe blow to
either of these two areas may cause damage all over the body but
mainly in the legs and back. The spine originally forms as a jellylike mass that eventually rounds itself into a hollow tube running
the length of the back. Another layer is then formed encasing the
first tube. A third layer is formed like a skin to protect everything
else. Out of this eventually come the bones (vertebrae) which
make up the spinal column. The illustrations show three vertebrae
from different sections of the spine (Fig. 2-11).
   The spine or vertebral column is made up of thirty-three segments joined by masses of tissue acting as cushions to allow movement and bending. The bones are kept apart but joined together
with strands of ligaments. As a person ages, the bone or cartilage
of the spine may become calcified or solid, restricting bending and

*The spinal column
is made up of
thirty-three segments,
called vertebrae.
They are joined by
strands of ligaments
and cushioned
so that they are
kept apart to
allow movement.*

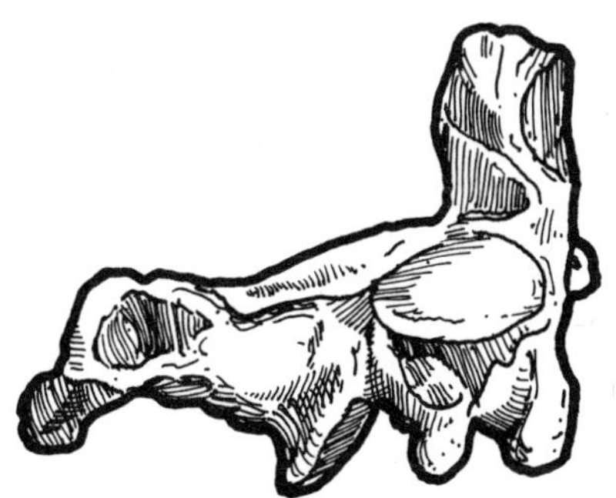

SECOND CERVICAL VERTEBRA

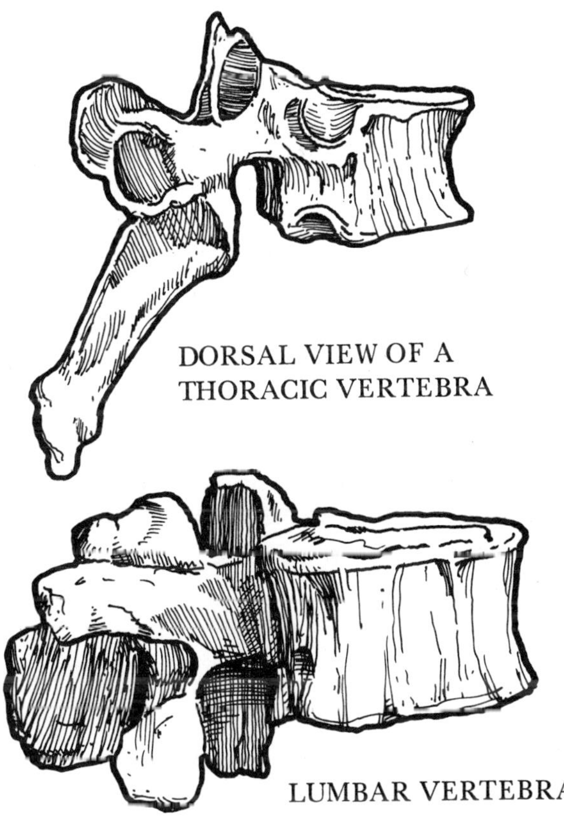

DORSAL VIEW OF A
THORACIC VERTEBRA

LUMBAR VERTEBRA

Figure 2 11

movement. The very small amount of fluid in these areas to begin with tends to dry up and harden. These bones don't have nerve endings in their basic make-up so when trouble begins, it is usually in the form of a stiffening of the back as opposed to pain. Over one quarter of the spine is made up of these discs or vertebrae, and they must maintain a good fluid balance for as long as possible in order to allow the spine to function properly. A good daily intake of fluid is recommended, along with proper exercising, in order to retain proper movement without restriction. This also helps the flow of oxygen and "food" throughout the spine. (Fig. 2-12).

In the course of your lifetime, the vertebrae become flattened down on top of one another, and movement is restricted. Sometimes, simply twisting or bending will cause the spine to "crack." The first fear is that something inside has snapped. In reality, the vertebrae were merely yanked apart, and the cracking was due to this. This may happen as often as once a week. It lets you know just how acute this settling process of the spine is.

The spinal disc, besides being a shock absorber, is also a mechanical structure with many functions. It allows for movement both up and down, forward and back, or any combination thereof. These discs are held together by strands of ligaments. The longer ones play a large part in the movement of the body while the shorter ones that join the discs at the sides are like a fixed webbing to hold each disc in place and keep them properly separated from each other. The spine distributes the weight evenly over the body. It is important to realize that the body doesn't have the whole weight to support directly, but the *distribution* of the force, allowing each section of the body to support only that part which it is supposed to. When the spine has a defective vertebra, it tends to pull the whole body to one side because of the strain on the ligaments, cords, and muscles. Then balance is lost.

The spine is like a protective wrapping around a tunnel that

*With age, these bones may become calcified
or flattened down on top of one another,
and movement is restricted.
Proper exercise and a good daily intake
of fluid is recommended.*

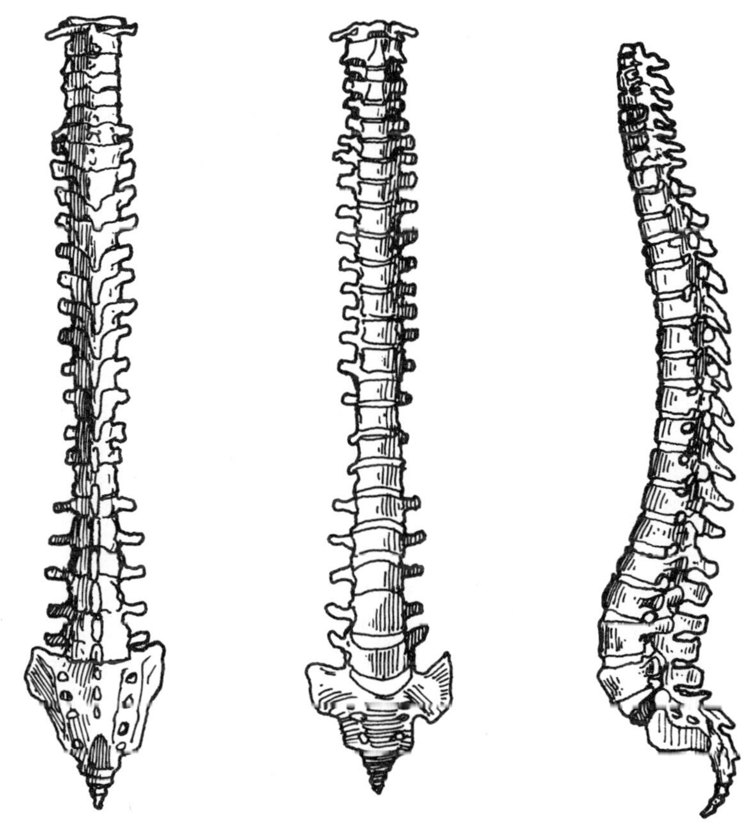

Figure 2-12   THREE VIEWS OF THE SPINAL COLUMN

holds the central nervous system of the whole body. When anything goes wrong in this area, the pains or aches we usually feel are coming from the central nervous system. In most whiplash accidents, the vertebrae are thrown out of place, and the result is a pinching of the nerve cord. When rolfing the spine, the palm of the hand or the elbow is placed in a position so that the vertebrae of the patient are spread apart, and the vertebral disc is forced back into its proper position. Immediate relief is felt.

There are two main curves or arcs in the spine. One is in the lower back and is the only one at birth, and the other is near the top of the neck. It develops in later years as the body matures. They are completely adaptable to twisting, turning, adjusting to, and countering just about all normal movement of the torso. Only under extreme strain or pressure will the body not be able to handle the situation, and this is the point at which damage occurs.

A total of seven vertebrae form the neck, and four variations are involved. The bone that sits over the top vertebra is like a ring allowing the head to rotate in a 180-degree arc without affecting the rest of the spine. In the mid-section the vertebrae are further apart, allowing the cords, ligaments, and muscles of the back to join but still have extensive play in them. What is seen as a hump in the back appears as if the neck is craning forward when, in reality, the neck is merely trying to keep a straight alignment with the waist and the feet. Close scrutiny will reveal this as in these illustrations (Fig. 2-13). When this person is rolfed or physically re-aligned, the hump disappears.

The dorsal and lumbar vertebrae differ in their slant and size. This allows for the natural curve seen in the spine. The smaller ones at the top are located where the rib cage is attached to the body. They are the weakest and, therefore, support the smaller and lighter ribs. The web of spinous cords hold, support, and control movement in the spine, and any vertebra that shifts out of position may cause a disruption in the whole spine, as well as placing a strain on the psoas muscles. These muscles are not designed

The neck appears to be craning forward,
and there is a hump in the back before rolfing.
After alignment with the waist and feet,
the hump disappears.

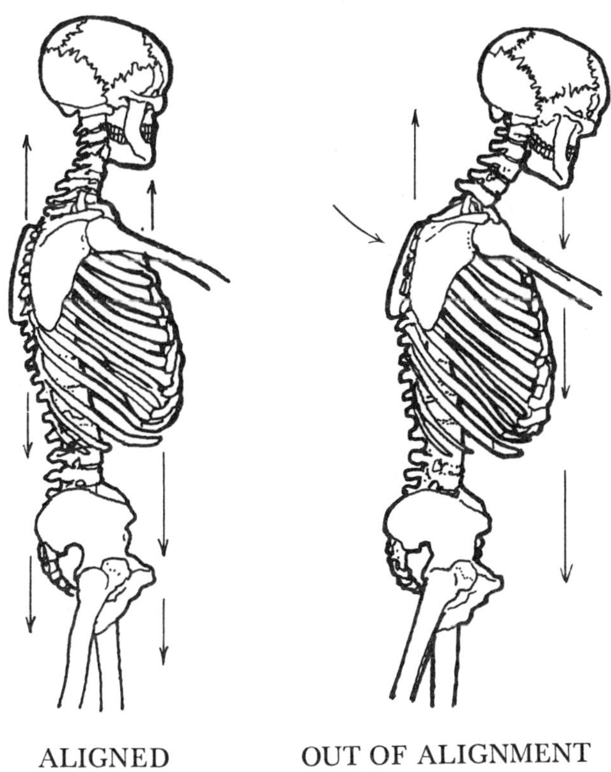

Figure 2-13

to take on another job, and relying on this compensation will only cause some form of permanent damage.

People who are virtually free of spinal problems seem to glide along when they walk, but the opposite is true of those who have something wrong. They walk with a trudging gait and never seem elated and happy. Everything they do is a chore, and they never feel like doing anything more than is necessary.

The nervous system is designed to do its best work in its natural and uninterrupted surroundings. It affects the whole person, and though the art of rolfing is not involved with the nervous system, it must be looked after. When an individual goes through a complete rolfing, the end result is almost total freedom in his skeletal structure so that it may perform properly and keep a balance with the gravitational pull downward. Remember, people deteriorate so slowly that they are unaware of it. They tend to feel normal. They have no idea how relaxed they would feel and how changed, both physically and mentally, along with their whole outlook on life.

Chapter 3

MOVEMENT

The body is never still but is in continuous motion. Even when someone appears to be still, he is still in motion trying to maintain balance. In breathing, the body is in motion from the pelvic region up to the head. Any movement, no matter how slight, involves a psychological movement of thoughts which, in turn, creates a different type of motion that most people are usually not consciously aware of. This is why, when treating anyone for a physical disorder, the physician should consider the mind, especially if the disorder is disrupting the patient's lifestyle or normal behavior patterns.

THE PULLEYS OF THE BODY

All humans from birth onward possess the ability to move, no matter how slight. This is all made possible through the system or network of pulleys and joints working together properly. Movement in the body is totally due to the workings of the muscles, tendons, ligaments, and cords, and sometimes when bone placement must be corrected through rolfing, the rolfer must first release the cords which have been "glued" to the bone structure because of overuse or lack of use. These cords then bind and restrict normal movement and can affect us at any age. Usually, it is due to a buildup over a period of time, and this buildup is so gradual that it goes unnoticed until a part of us just stops working. This is when panic sets in, and professional help is sought to correct the problem.

As babies, we have the natural ability to move without thought, even though we are not in control of our limbs as yet. Noticing the hands move is usually the first step in the realization that we have them. It is the movement that attracts the eye.

The feet are next and usually become playthings. Crawling, sitting, standing, and walking are usually not possible until the ages of six to nine months in order for the working pulleys of the body to gain strength and balance.

Sitting becomes a natural urge, and this is actually where the baby's first sense of balance comes into play, and weight is settled over the pelvic area for the first time. When the child begins to crawl, the knee joints receive their first attempt at weight distribution. These are important times in the development of the child, and the parents should guide and assist him.

The development of bad habits should be noticed immediately and corrected because this is where the frame is most easily damaged. Every section of the bone structure has not had the time to develop to its fullest strength. The size of the muscles and cords of the baby's legs are proportionate to the size of the leg but not always to the weight. When this problem exists, then the muscles in the legs must work overtime.

The corrective measures in rolfing children are to work the muscles which are affecting the joints and to soften them until their hold on the joint is released. Then the joints are twisted back into position. This can be a little painful, depending upon the extent of the damaged area. Once the treatment is finished, the child must be exercised but kept off his feet until sufficient strength is developed to support the weight of the body.

If the same condition is found in a mature adult, it has usually been in existence for a period of time, and the joints have probably suffered severe damage. He most likely refers to the aches and pains of his condition as arthritis or rheumatism. The same treatment is followed, but relief of the situation may take longer or may not be completely effective.

JOINTS

All movement in the body is determined by the proper functioning of the joints. Whether they are large bony masses or small in-

terlocking pieces, the joints are held together by fibrous cartilage
acting as a joining substance to hold one bone to another and as
a cushion to evenly distribute the weight being brought down
upon the bones from the normal downward gravitational pull of
the earth. This is very obvious in the joining of the vertebrae in
the spinal column. Here the discs are separated by a spongy cushion of jellylike fluid that works as a shock absorber upon which
each disc relies. If this column has been damaged by too much
twisting or downward pressure, the strain on its outer wall will
cause a herniated disc. This forms a bulge in the outer wall, like
a strong rubberband holding the discs together instead of apart.
The result is great pain in most movement, especially in bending
or twisting.

Some of our joints are very small but are joined in much the
same manner and can be damaged just like a larger one. The larger joints, which are referred to as ball and socket joints, are protected by a complete circle of fibro-cartilage. They allow us a
greater amount of movement in areas such as the knees, elbows,
hips, and shoulders (Fig. 3-1).

Joints are usually thought of as just part of the bone mass. In
reality, they play a much more important part in that they join
two bone structures, are stretchable in their ability to lengthen
and shorten with movement, and they become a cushion, keeping
the two sections of bone from colliding with each other. If there
is any malfunction in the area that holds the joints apart, then
there is a problem, no matter how slight, in movement. Usually
we compensate for this by counterbalancing which, in turn, puts
added pressure on another area. This does not always show up as
a direct strain but causes fatigue or may show up as a dull pain and
aching joints. In movement, there is always a combination of ef-
forts by more than one joint, and when one is affected, the others
are affected as well. This is a direct leak of energy.

An unhealthy look, coupled with a tired, drawnout feeling,
makes us feel worse than we actually are. After rolfing treatment,
which begins with the feet, the waist and pelvic area become better balanced. Improved posture and a more relaxed feeling are the

The joints are held together by fibrous cartilage.
Larger joints are referred to as "ball and socket"
joints and allow us a greater amount
of movement in areas such as the elbows.
A damaged joint causes great pain.

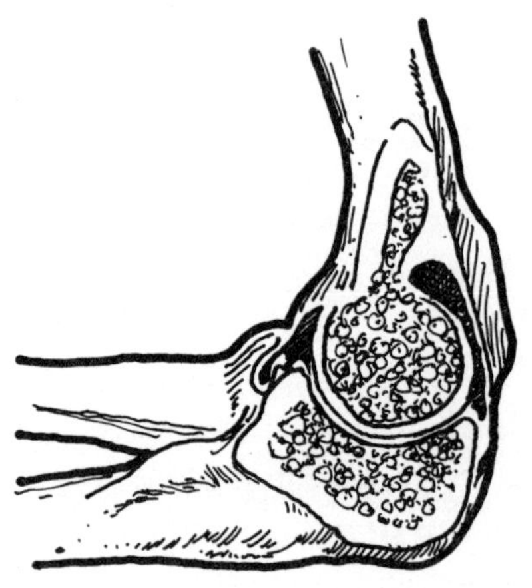

INTERNAL VIEW OF ELBOW JOINT

Figure 3-1

immediate results (Fig. 3-2).

THE MUSCLES

Muscles act as strong cables, working the joints, and allowing us movement. Some are extremely small with very small but important jobs while others are massive and cause major problems if damaged. Almost all of the major muscles of the body run up and down, the same way as the bones do. They become pulled or strained, tired and overworked, twisted or even cut in a severe accident. Whatever the case may be, whenever anyone has a muscle affected to the point of damage, then immobility may result.

Some muscles hold pieces of bone in place, with one pulling and working in one direction while another counterbalances in the opposite direction. When one is hurt, the other may try to take over the work of both, which then leads to strain.

Muscles also act as power units allowing us to run for long distances, perform heavy work, and accept blows. When a muscle is struck, no matter how, its natural reaction is to constrict. The reaction is pain or stiffening of the part which was damaged. This means immobility. The quickest way to relieve this tension is to exercise the area, either directly, or through manipulation of the muscle. This begins an immediate relaxation of the muscle and starts it on its journey back to performing its proper function in the body.

In the iliac region, the *psoas* muscle acts in conjunction with the *iliacus* and the *pyriformis* muscles as a major contracting and stretching band between the pelvis and the thigh during walking. They share a common linkup with the femur or hip bone. The three muscles — the psoas, the iliacus, and the pyriformis — are the muscle web connected to the sacrum and play a large role in maintaining the upright and straight structural alignment of the spinal column. Therefore if the chemistry is upset or any other disorder occurs, the whole balance of the structure is changed. Through proper structural realignment, they may be disentangled and reset into proper working order. All these muscles play a part

*Rolfing treatment begins with the feet
and continues up to the waist and pelvic area.
The immediate results are improved posture
and a less tired, more relaxed feeling.*

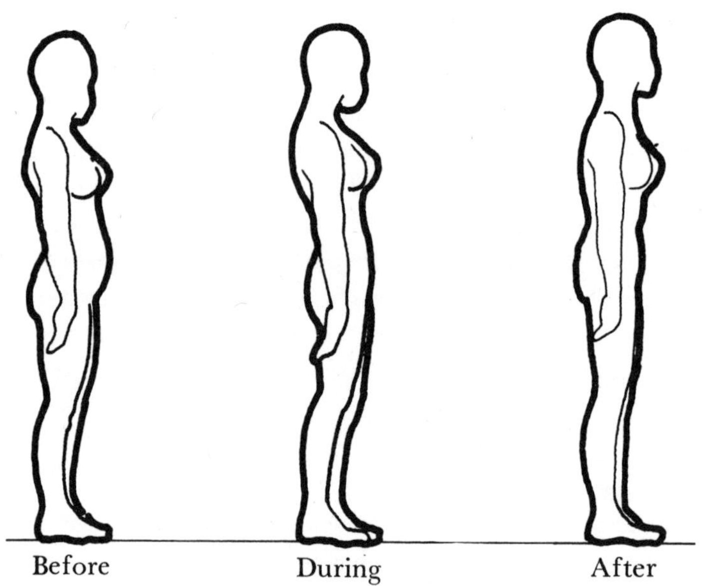

RESULTS OF ROLFING

Figure 3-2

in the flexibility and rotation of the pelvic region or waist area.
If, in most cases, the rectus femoris takes over to compensate for
a damaged or pulled area, then the psoas muscle ceases to function and begins to deteriorate. When this happens and these other muscles begin to do the work of the psoas, then the lumbar
function is impeded. The result is usually severe dull backache
(Fig. 3-3).

The *hamstrings*, small muscles joined along the bottom of the
pelvic bone, balloon out into a blanket of muscle covering about
.2 percent of the thigh area. They run down the leg together for
about three-quarters of the way and then spread out to attach
themselves, two on the inner side of the leg below the knee, and
one on the outer side. If they shorten, it creates a downward tug
in the pelvic area and tilts the pelvis forward and down. This creates problems in the weight distribution over the pelvic basin,
down to the knee and ankle joints; and in the top half of the torso, the base of the back sits unbalanced over the whole structure.
The only way the problem may be corrected is by lengthening the
hamstrings to take the pull off the pelvis and allow it to tilt back
up to its proper position.

The *sartorius* muscle, the longest muscle in the body, comes
from the back of the pelvic structure, wraps around and down the
thigh to attach itself behind the leg and below the knee. It is in-
terwoven with the hamstring muscles, and if it is shortened, it may
throw the whole knee joint into rotation, causing the rest of the
pelvic and thigh muscles to twist out of position.

Irregular sitting habits and various types of exercises may lead
to shortening of the sartorius muscle to the extent of causing a
rotation in the whole pelvis. It means that the shortening has
caused such a strong pull that the counter-pulling muscle has lost
its effectiveness and can no longer keep things evenly balanced.
A person with this overpull in the sartorius muscle will appear to
be standing straight, but there is a definite twist in the hips.

In the thigh area of the human body, there are many muscles.
Some shorten in length with movement while others lengthen.
There are four main muscles in the inner thigh which run from
the base of the pelvic structure to different points along the inner

The muscles in the iliac region
play a part in the flexibility and rotation
of the pelvic area.
If one of these muscles is damaged or pulled,
the result is severe, dull backache.

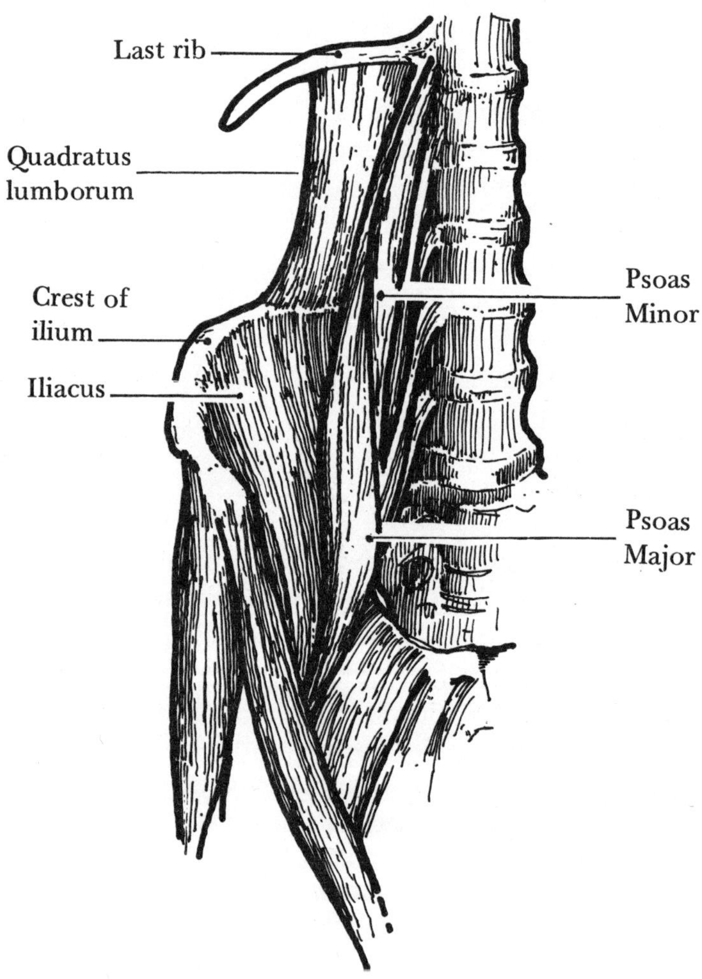

Figure 3-3

thigh bone. There is one tensor muscle that extends from the up-per outside of the pelvis to the outside of the tibia below the knee joint. From the back to the front, there are three main muscles called the *vastus lateralis,* the *rectus femoris,* and the *vastus medi-alis.* These muscles in the thigh area control the proper upright position of the pelvis and control complete movement in this area which, in turn, affects the whole movement of the legs (Fig. 3-4).

These three muscles, located in the back of the thigh, extend down to attach to the top of the tibia below the kneecap. Since a child does not begin to use these muscles in the legs until he or she begins to crawl, stand, or walk, problems don't usually show up until three to five years of age. A defect is easily noticed but sometimes is neglected, and this only creates larger and more dif-ficult problems.

Due to the flexibility of a child's bones and muscles, restructur-ing is much simpler, but when it involves an adult whose muscles have become tight, and the bones have settled into wrong posi-tions, then a longer period of time, sometimes more painful treat-ment, and the chance that the problem has gone too far are prob-able. Neglect is one of the biggest problems.

More complications exist in the gluteal area for this is the seat of movement within the human body. Weight distribution is all centered in this area, from the top of the head all the way down, and when this area is upset, then the total moving struc-ture is affected. The top of the body is disturbed due to the problem of balance. The bottom half, which causes the top half to be off balance, is disrupted because the weight is distri-buted unevenly, causing dislocations by rotation, overworked muscles, and pain.

Not counting the tendons, cords, and muscles which come from outside this area and attach themselves to the pelvis, there are two horizontal muscles: the *gluteus medius* and the *gluteus minimus* which have the job of pulling the pelvis into position with the upper thigh bone. Three other muscles which are later-al positioners are the *pyriformis,* the *obturator internus,* and the *quadratus femoris.* Their main job is to stabilize the positioning

*There are many muscles in the thigh
which control the proper upright position
of the pelvis. Some shorten in length
with movement while others lengthen.*

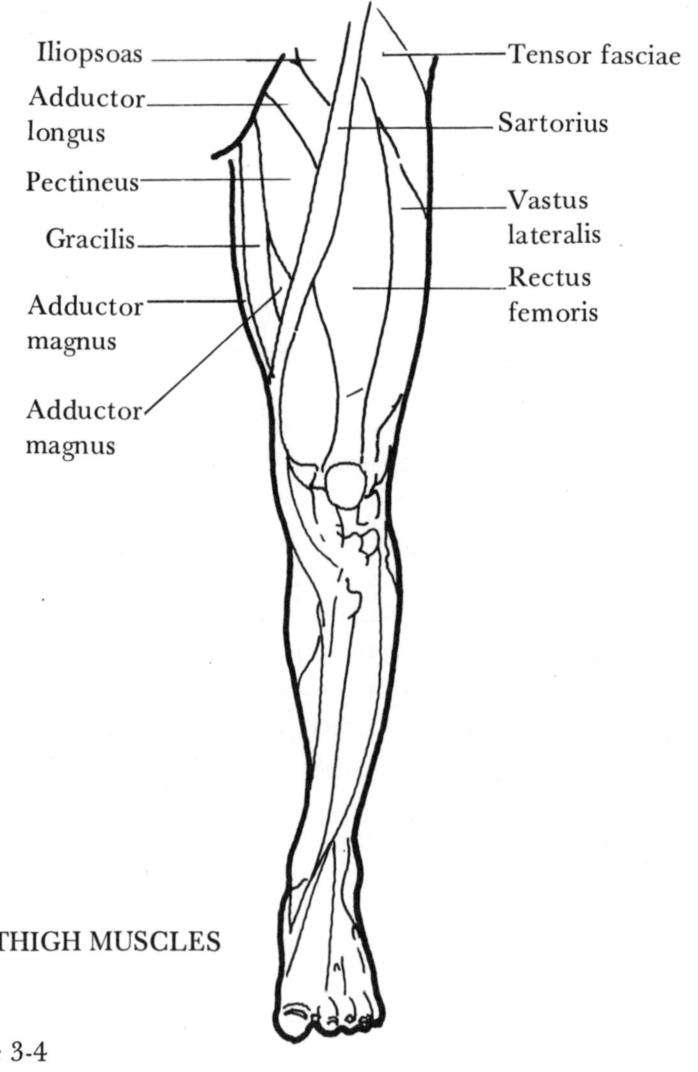

THIGH MUSCLES

Figure 3-4

of the pelvis over the lower area of the body. This combination of horizontal and lateral muscles is the main unit that makes sure the pelvis sits centrally over the rest of the body. This unit also controls the forward and backward movement of the pelvis, which we use mostly in sitting or getting up.

When any one of these inner or outer muscles is damaged due to overwork, strain, or through bone dislocation, then there is a distinct change in gait, and if it is not seen to immediately, greater damage will undoubtedly occur.

In order to correct any damage in this area, a patient must be as relaxed as possible, which isn't easy, and the rolfer must use a great amount of force in resituating these affected regions. If the main tensor muscle that runs from the principal front thigh muscle up to the front and top of the pelvis is struck or overworked, then it shortens, and because it has direct relation to the gluteus medius and minimus through a nerve system, then all areas are affected, not just the main tensor muscle.

When the pelvic area is in need of structural alignment, it usually means that the upper part of the torso has been disturbed. This results in difficulty of movement and also has a distinct effect on the nervous system. Any restrictions or tension in the body creates an uncomfortable situation, and the patient has difficulty sleeping and is usually tense in living day to day.

The upper part of the leg that is connected to the pelvis consists of many muscles. They play a most important part in holding the pelvis in position. They are connected to the pelvic basin on the inner part of the thigh. Their main importance is to keep the pelvis in correct vertical and horizontal position.

Most people aren't aware of muscles existing in the feet. We are more aware, however, of the muscles existing in the backs or calves of our legs for these become painful when we are overtired. The bulky portion of the leg is made up of muscle tissue, both protecting the leg and giving it strength. From the knee down, there are four main muscles controlling the leg. They are the right and left *gastrocnemius* and the right and left *soleus* muscles. The knee joint is made of the bone mass, ligaments, and tendons (Fig. 3-5).

Fig. 3-5

Most people are very aware of the muscles in the backs or calves of their legs for they become painful when they are overtired. Muscle tissue makes up the bulk of the leg, both protecting it and giving it strength.

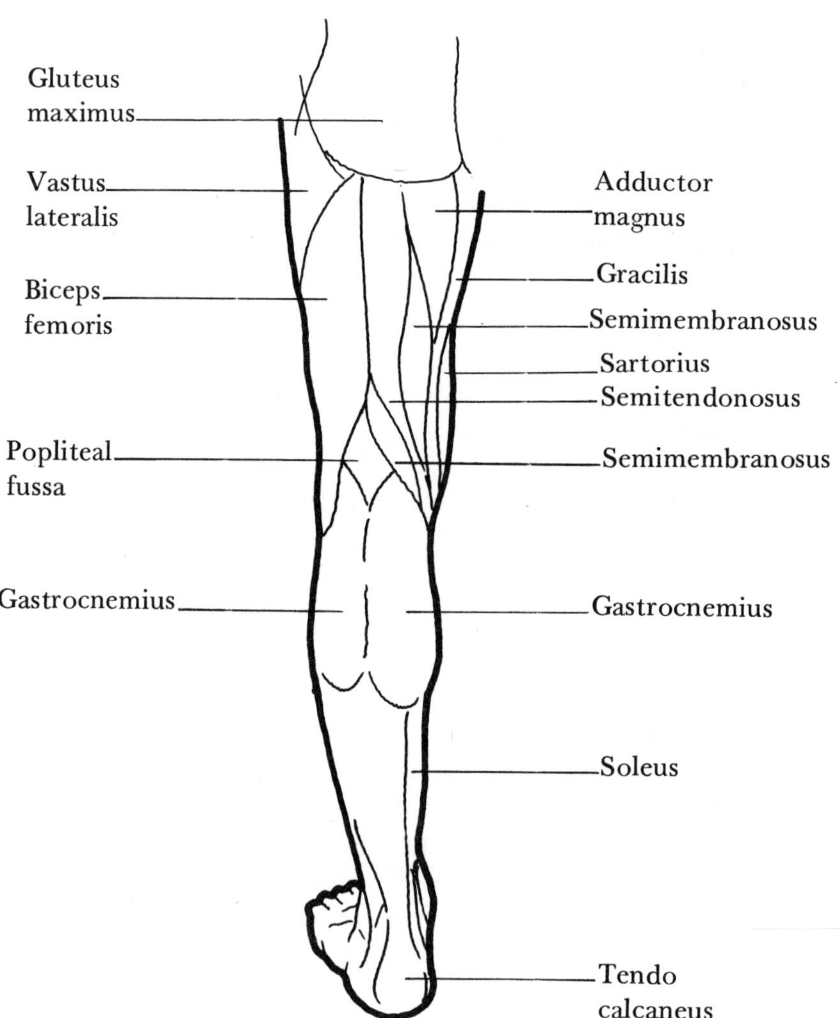

Figure 3-5

As we enter the pelvis and upper torso, we must approach the rolfing treatment in a much stronger manner because we are dealing with deep, internally situated muscles and bone structure that take a while to correct and can cause some pain in the process.

The torso has both inner and outer important, controlling muscles that may be easily damaged through physical abuse or from overstraining which may occur when the skeletal structure is out of alignment. All muscles in the body are important, but the main causes for concern are the *quadratus lumborum,* the *psoas major,* the *psoas minor,* and the *rectus abdominis* which are the back muscles running up and down on either side of the spinal column. The chief function of these muscles is to help maintain correct posture (Figs. 3-3 and 3-6).

The back, leading up to the neck area, is encased in a network of muscles which interlock and cross back and forth over it, both protecting and adding physical support. There are about a dozen of these, and the whole mass is enclosed in another wrapping of muscle called the *trapezius* muscle. Each has its own part in the distribution of the work, as well as assisting one another if one is damaged. They play an important role in keeping the entire upper structure balanced in a central position (Fig. 3-7).

In the shoulder there are about five main controlling muscles which play an important part in the movement of the arms. They are the *deltoid, biceps brachii, coraco-brachialis, latissimus dorsi,* and the *pectoralis major* (Fig. 3-8). They get daily exercise almost from birth. Problems in this area are usually very rare unless there is a birth defect. These muscles begin to strengthen almost immediately and continue to grow stronger with the growth of the child. The underlying set of muscles and cords do their part along with the outer ones in holding the bone structure in place and allowing it freedom of movement. However, if any one of these should tighten or shorten through injury or overstrain due to lifting excess amounts of weight, then the humerus joint at the top of the shoulder may become twisted and pulled. The whole arm is affected and probably a great deal of the shoulder going up as far as the neck. This is very common in athletes,

Some of the muscles in the torso that help maintain correct posture may become easily damaged through physical abuse or from overstraining.

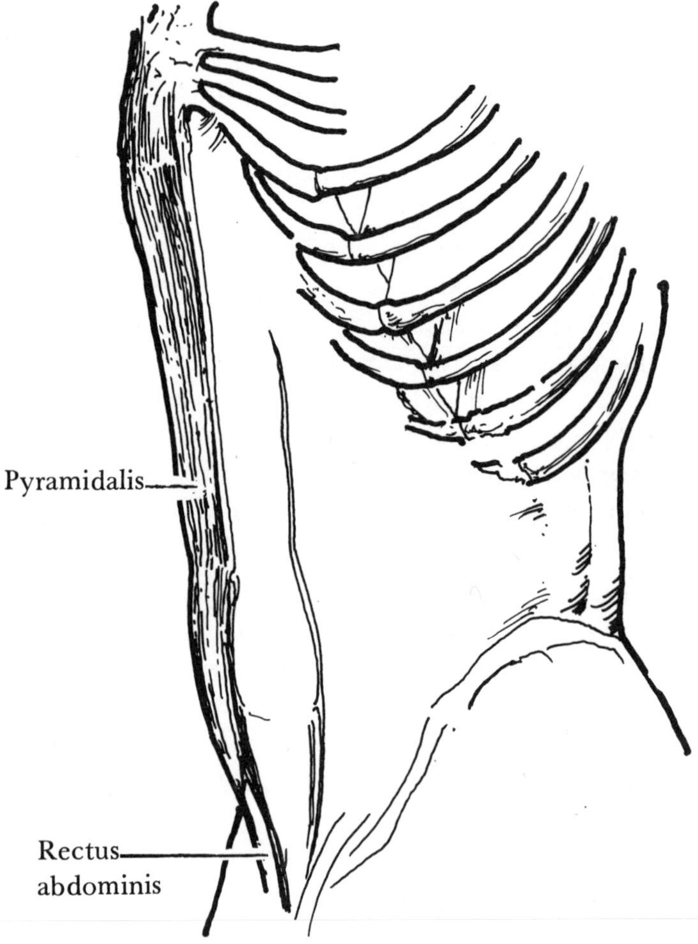

Figure 3-6

*A network of muscles encases the back,
protecting it and adding physical support.
These muscles interlock, cross back and forth,
and assist one another.*

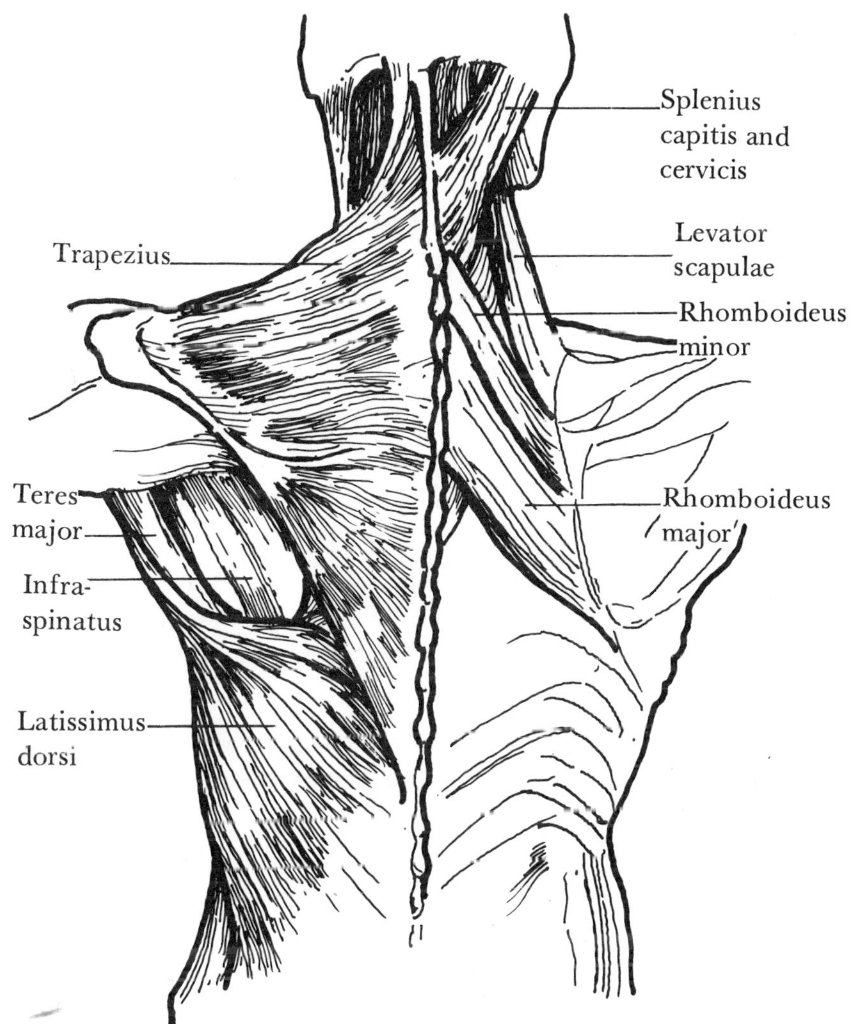

Figure 3-7

The controlling muscles which play an important part in the movement of the arms get daily exercise almost from birth. They strengthen immediately and rarely cause any problems. However, injuries are common among athletes, especially in contact sports.

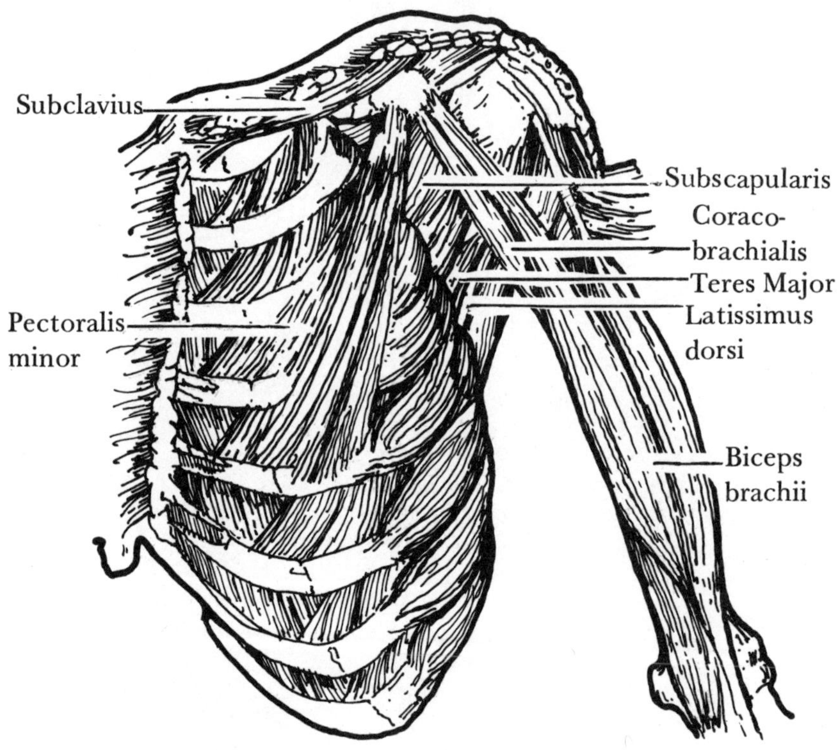

Figure 3-8   SHOULDER AND ARM PULLEYS

Flexor muscles that stretch and contract

allow the head to tilt from side to side.

Other muscles in the neck

hold the upper part of the spine erect

and control the counterbalancing of the head.

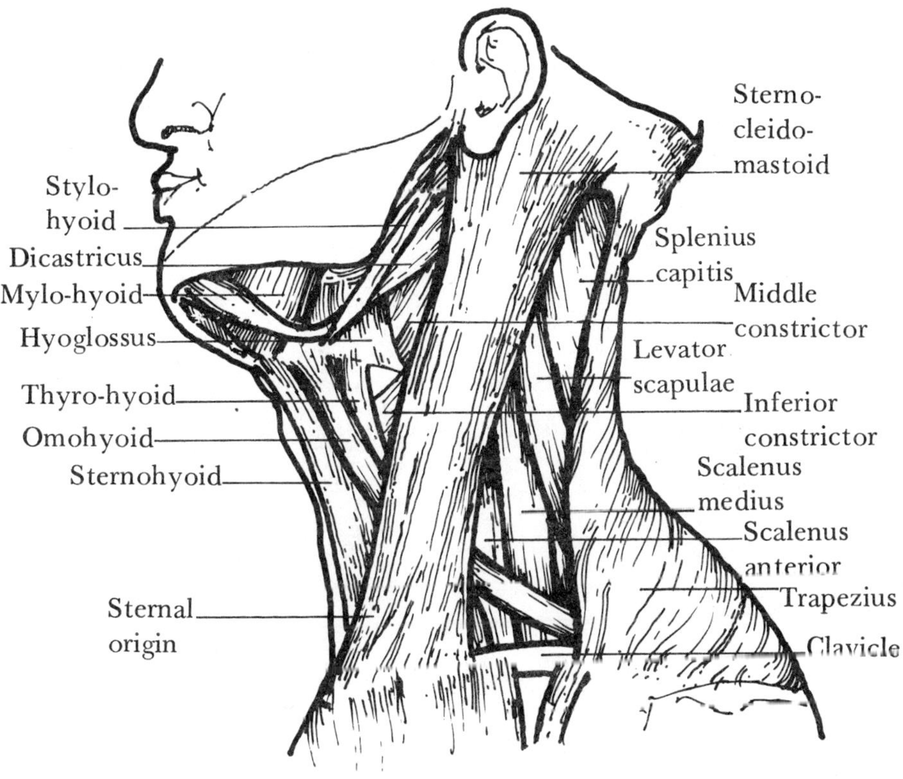

Figure 3-9

especially in contact sports.

The neck is supported by three main muscles, chiefly the *splenius capitis* which is referred to as the postvertebra muscle. This muscle holds the upper part of the spine erect while the *sterno-cleido-mastoid* muscle controls the counterbalancing of the head. Connected to the base of the skull, it runs or extends forward to attach to the top part of the first rib. The third is the *levator scapulae.*

Then there are three counterbalancing muscles which control the side movement of the head. They are called the *scalenus anterior, medius,* and *posterior* muscles or the front, middle, and back. They are flexor muscles that stretch and contract to allow the head to tilt from side to side. The front and middle muscles are joined to the first rib while the back muscles hook onto the second rib of the rib cage. They all run up and adjoin the first spinal vertebra (Fig. 3-9).

Chapter 4

THE UPPER TORSO

The main areas of the top half of the torso are the supporting back muscles, the neck, and the head. The upper part of the spinal column is related to the back and the shoulder girdle. When the arms and shoulders are overworked, the spine is badly affected. All of this upper section forms a machine that must work as a unit in order for each part to function properly.

THE SHOULDER GIRDLE

The shoulder girdle is balanced on the upper part of the body and held there by only one connection. The gravitational pull and its delicate position make it very vulnerable to damage. Any damage in this area leads to headaches, stiffness, and limited movement in the upper extremities. The pectoral and pelvic girdles play an important part in the total movement of the whole body. The psoas and the rhomboideus muscles connect the two bony girdles to the spine to work together as one unit of movement. Every part must be attached properly, yet be able to operate as a well-greased set of cables to allow the proper moving ability. The rhomboideus set of muscles controls the mobility of the shoulder girdle while the psoas muscles reign over the pelvic girdle. The center of these working muscle units comes together in the lumbo-dorsal junction.

The shoulder blade, called the *scapula*, is attached to the five upper, outer ribs by muscles. It has a certain amount of flexibility but remains in place. The humerus, or upper arm bone, is fitted into a cuplike joint on the outside of the scapula and is held together with small muscles and cartilage. A large piece of cartilage joins the unit to the front of the rib cage. Each of the muscles involved in the shoulder joint stretches and relaxes in order to allow maximum movement without any restraint (Fig. 4-1).

The *clavicles* or collarbones are found in front, running inward from the shoulders to the center of the chest (sternum). These act as a support in keeping the body upright. The first and second ribs aid in support, under the collarbones, and help keep the shoulders in alignment.

The clavicles determine the distance between the shoulders and the flexibility of the arms, in general. If the scapula or the shoulder socket for the humerus is pushed too far back toward the spine, it will show as an indentation along the spine and the shoulder blades will protrude in back. Should the collarbone become stuck or molded to the top rib of the rib cage, a noticeable stoop results, along with a dragging gait. This gives a humped look to the upper spine and causes pain in the lower back because of the strain.

The *humerus* or top part of the arm is joined to the main part of the body by large and small muscles. If the rhomboideus muscles are in proper perspective to the bone structure, then proper movement will result. If not, the collarbone will ride too high, and the back blades will move too freely. If the muscle tone is not right, it will affect either the over- or underlying muscles and cause either restriction or too much movement.

The upper part of the dorsal scapula plays an important part in protecting the humerus while it is locked in the socket cup. It also controls the upward stretch of the arm. If it is working properly without any restriction, then the arm will usually have unlimited movement. The muscles connecting the upper arm to the scapula are very flexible and usually allow much freedom of movement. This also exposes them to disruption very easily which then automatically restrains movement in the arm. When this happens, the top part of the arm bone becomes encased in the muscles as if lying in a hammock. Then the rib cage is affected with every movement, and respiratory and cardiac problems could eventually arise.

The delicate position of the shoulder girdle
makes it very vulnerable to damage.
Each part must work properly to allow maximum
movement without restraint. If any part of the unit
is hurt, it will affect motion in the upper limbs.

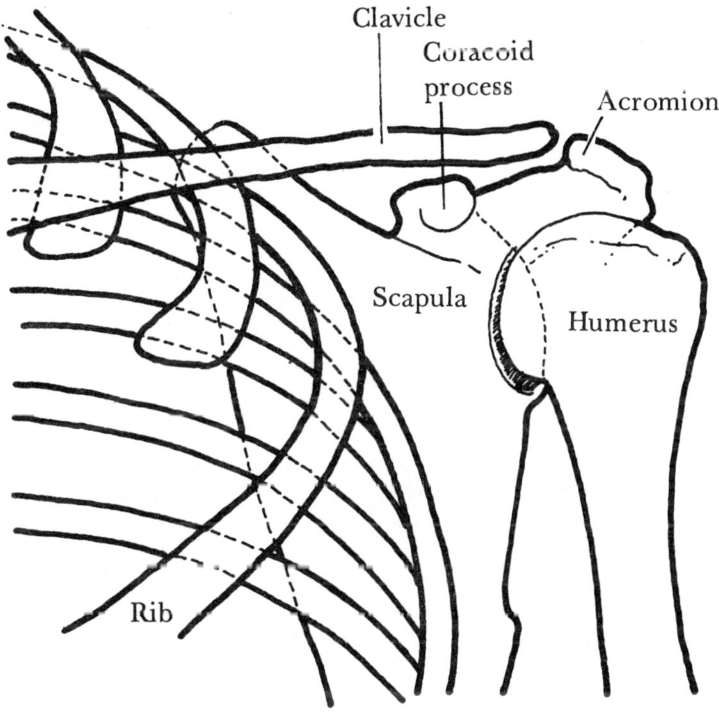

Figure 4-1

The shoulder girdle, sitting on top of the whole torso, controls the movement in the upper limbs. If any one part of this working mechanism is disrupted, then the whole unit is affected. It may not always stop working altogether, but it will slow down and have a direct effect on some other part, namely the rib cage. Some questions are presented here for you to check your shoulder area. When standing upright or sitting properly, is there any discomfort in the shoulder or the neck? Is there adequate freedom of movement? The arms and the shoulders should move freely without any help from the spine and no twisting of the body. While standing, see if you are able to lift the torso of the body by stretching upwards. The shoulders and head should not move up with this action but should remain fairly stable. If this is possible then the rhomboideus muscles are in good working order.

Observe the horizontal line drawn from one shoulder across to the other. Keep your eyes on the collarbones or clavicles. If they are functioning properly, then the shoulders will seem to be evenly aligned. If one shoulder is lower or higher than the other, there is a definite strain from somewhere else, and a problem exists.

THE ART OF BEING UPRIGHT

In order for the human body to function properly and maintain an upright position, five basic points of the body must be in alignment. These five main points are: the central point of the ear, the shoulder joint, the hip joint, the knee joint, and the ankle joint. The head, neck, and shoulders tell the story of the structure below them. In the East, they say that a man should carry himself as if he were suspended in the air by an imaginary rope holding him upright by the hair. The body should glide along, rather than look as if it has to do extremely hard work with every step it takes. The head and neck must be centered over the middle of the body, and the spine that supports the structure must be at the back of the pelvic section. The spine must then curve in conjunction with the natural back curvature until it enters the base of the skull in a central direction. Any damage or constant pressure will disturb the balance of the upper torso.

The head and neck, along with the shoulders, work as a unit controlled by four main working muscles. They are the *sterno-cleido-mastoid, levator scapula, trapezius,* and *splenius* muscles. They are support muscles, rather than actual laboring muscles. When a neck problem exists, these muscles take over in controlling movement from the shoulder where they are attached.

There are two main arteries that are important in the neck area. The *carotid* artery carries blood and other important food nutrients to the head which encases the brain. The *vertebral* artery carries the much needed food through to the vertebrae of the spine. Any disruption of the flow to this area causes immediate trouble. The carotid artery, because it travels to the brain, must have free access in its route. Any impediment will not only deprive the head of the food it needs, but will also cut off the blood and oxygen supply to the brain, resulting in a faint.

In the spine where the vertebral artery passes through, a pure uninterrupted flow must exist. Any dislodging of the vertebrae will pinch the tube carrying the all-important food. Whiplash is one of the greatest hazards in which this takes place. If the head is tilted forward, and a cutoff of the flow of body food results, there is also a slowdown in oxygen and blood supply. This will cause both physical and mental impairment.

In younger people, when circulation is interrupted, it is usually felt in the form of a sharp pain in the neck and upper back area. This is the nerve's way of telling us that something is wrong and should be cared for immediately.

The *cranium* should sit in a balanced position on top of the rest of the body. It usually tilts forward slightly. A series of three muscles is involved in the even balancing of the head. These muscles normally are not seen. When a person seems to be cowering or shrugging his shoulders, it is the result of a shortening of the muscles that hold the neck and head in their proper position. These muscles have a tendency to tighten which causes the shoulder blades to adhere to the trapezius muscle. It automatically brings on a severe loss of bending movement and causes the dorsal vertebrae and ribs to bunch tightly together.

When rolfing techniques are applied to the tight areas and the muscles allowed to move freely once more, the vertebrae and the ribs return to their proper positions, and the strain is taken off those parts used to compensate for the restricted muscles (Fig. 4-2).

THE NECK

The longer muscles that help in the upright support of the neck are at the base of the skull. They make up the bulk of the mass which we know as "neck." As they proceed down the dorsal vertebrae of the spinal column, they spread out and form a webbing of muscles which attach to different vertebrae. Neck pains and upper or lower backaches are usually caused by lack of flexibility in these sets of muscles. When the muscles harden and rest on the spine over a period of time, they drastically restrict natural body movement. In treating this, the rolfer applies pressure, both up and down, to help replace these muscles in their normal positions and restore their elasticity. Almost immediately after, the person receiving the rolfing treatment feels relief, even though during the actual treatment he may feel extreme pain or discomfort.

Due to the relationship and dependence of one part of the body on another, any damage that may exist, even in the extremities, affects the neck and head.

THE HEAD

We are now at the top of the human structure, the hood of knowledge. The central force in our mobility is the waist or pelvic region, supporting the thorax of the body. It is an amazing structure that cannot function without a thinking unit to direct it. This thinking unit, encased in the head or skull, is a telegraph system, sending messages to all parts of our bodies and telling them

*When muscles tighten, they cause
not only pain but a loss of bending movement.
Rolfing techniques, applied to the tight areas,
allow the muscles to move freely once more,
and the vertebrae and ribs
return to their proper positions.*

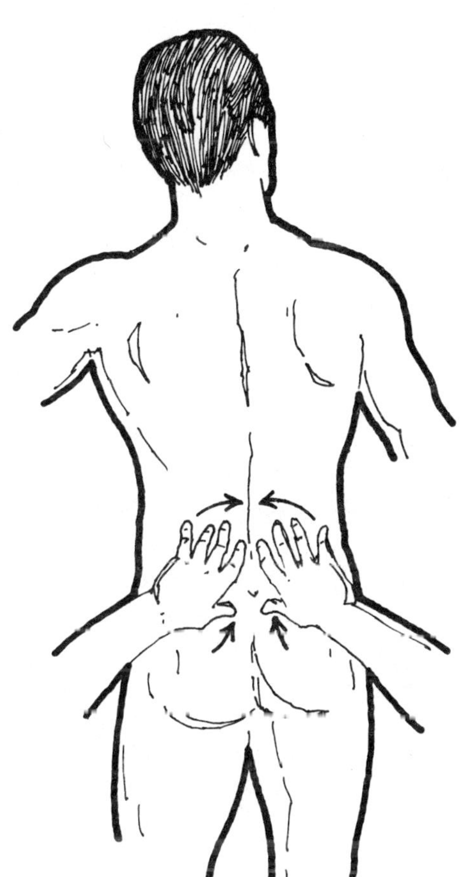

Figure 4-2

what to do. Exactly what is this head, what is it made up of, and what are its functions and malfunctions?

The cranium is the case in which the brain is situated. The brain is the most intricate part of the nervous system. At birth the head or skull is made up of a series of small bony segments which in later life grow and join together as one piece, the skull. In newborn children, the brain is protected only by a membrane, the "soft spot."

The feet, the pelvis, and the head all relate to one another in trying to keep aligned, one above the other. Take a good look at a picture of a man or a woman standing in a fixed position and see if you are able to spot this.

The muscles at the back of the neck allow you to nod forward and to pull the head back into position. When the head is thrown off balance, manipulation of these head and neck muscles will aid in the restoration of this balance.

Besides being a mass of large segments of bone, the head also contains its share of smaller ones that are very delicately placed. There are two large bones which expand and contract in order that the head may absorb the shock resulting from a blow or jolt. The *sphenoid* bone, which resembles a bat with its wings spread, is the segment that helps keep the walls of the skull in their proper perspective. There are a total of eight bones in the cranial cavity and fourteen bones in the facial part of the head. When cartilages and muscles become strained due to overwork, then this strain is felt all the way through the body to the head. The upper back, neck, and head are all interacting in the sense that if one or all are affected by any disorder, the mind is also affected. If only one of these areas is out of balance, it will affect them all.

Sometimes certain jobs require an individual to be in one position for a long period of time. This almost certainly has an effect. Blows to the side of the head, whether accidental or from a profession such as boxing, alter the position of the sphenoid bone and cause a disruption of the optical nerve cords.

In the eye itself, there is a total of six muscles. Four control the up-and-down movement of the eye and two control the side-to-side movement.

When the muscles in the head are relaxed, they are all capable of doing their proper functions. Any strain, no matter what the cause, may force these muscles to constrict. This, in turn, affects the rest of the muscles due to the overwork or strain placed on them.

Chapter 5

THE HUMAN RESPONSE

More and more we are becoming acutely aware of pain because we are not used to hard work or hardships of the kind our forebears knew. We move in an almost automated society where most of the tedious chores are done for us with the push of a button.

Pain comes in many forms, the most common being physical, with emotional or psychological pain following. We are creatures of habit and do not easily bend to change. When we are forced to change we automatically become leary of it. As we mature, we overcome these fears to some extent but never really lose them. Fear is merely a reaction to the unknown. It is natural to be afraid of the unknown and only the fool is not. That which is painful to one individual may be nothing to another. Fear is triggered by our nervous systems, and we have no control over this highly sensitive reaction in our bodies.

In the field of medicine, we frequently wait until the last minute to have a disorder in our bodies looked into for fear that it is something fatal when most of the time, it is easily cured. People are simply afraid to admit that there is something wrong. Even from childhood we are brainwashed into a fear of doctors and dentists. This fear can only be overcome through education, explaining the unknown. I have always been in favor of lecturing and public speaking on the part of a cancer patient or someone who has been crippled by a disease and has overcome the mental and physical handicaps that inevitably accompany it. This is education, and it will help overcome fears in the world we live in. Any practice that is unheard of in society is automatically feared or looked on with suspicion and apprehension because there is no information on it available to the public.

Our bodies feel normal to us even when they are in an abnormal state. This is because we have functioned this way for the better part of our existence, and we think that is normal. When something is wrong, we do our best to ignore the fact even though we are aware that it exists. When we are injured we acknowledge pain in varying degrees. In some people, there is almost no reaction while in others it is extreme.

Emotional pain shows up on the facial features as extreme anguish lines in the jowls, frowns in the lines above the eyebrows, and temperament to go along with this. All other strains show up in much the same way, in continual distress and in poor appearance.

If someone approaches a rolfer for treatment or evaluation, he is automatically afraid because it is an unknown. He may be helped to relax through conversation and explanation along with a demonstration of the art or profession of rolfing. Fear of the unknown can even turn into pain through a combination of psychological and emotional reactions which are simply devices for self-preservation.

Emotional pain is sometimes incorrectly taken care of by drugs, alcohol, or physical abuse. A nervous breakdown due to the lack of ability to handle the emotional strain may also result.

When pain is inflicted on humans, be it physical or emotional, there is always a response. When this response takes place, there is an actual physical change in the chemistry of the individual's system. This change disrupts body functions and causes a reaction. If the pain is physical, the damage causes pain in the immediate area of damage and then spreads to other areas.

In rolfing, we are simply stating that there exists a certain amount of natural damage in just about every human that is brought on by everyday living. This damage goes unnoticed because we become accustomed to it and feel as if it is normal. It reaches a point where we actually have no idea what feeling normal is really like. If we changed for the better, whether through the usual medical treatment, psychotherapy, or rolfing, we are

afraid and uncertain of the result because, basically, we don't know
how we are supposed to feel. It is again the unknown that we fear.

All forms of human response can be traced back to a physiological disorder or malfunction. Traumatic shock is brought on by a
physical force. We see physical responses, not internal responses.
When we are affected internally, we don't see it unless there is
some physical manifestation. Some people may become deaf,
lame, or blind as physical responses to some inner problem. Fear
can create this type of reaction.

Emotions — pain, joy, tranquility, sadness — are usually shown
in our facial features. We are unable to control it. In this way,
sickness is definitely portrayed through our features. A person
trained in the medical profession should be capable of seeing these
responses long before the average layman. Even the voice will
show signs of some problems.

Rolfing takes a look at both the inner and outer structure as a
whole and tries to combine them into one to create a machine
that is well oiled and in good working order.

The minute conception occurs, we begin to grow old and deteriorate. A malfunction may take place during pregnancy that will
affect our growth and health after we are born. If we are lucky
enough to come through this period safely, the next step is childhood. This is a very important stage in that so much damage may
happen if proper teaching methods aren't followed. Walking is the
first actual stage where weight has begun to put pressure on the
structural frame, and if its distribution isn't handled carefully, then
problems begin to develop from the start.

From birth up to the end of the first year, the child is cared for
and looked after by his parents, but after the first year, his bones
begin to harden, and the cords and muscles get stronger as he is
taught how to use his own motor sensors and starts to fend for
himself. By watching and imitating, he discovers his lower limbs
which hadn't been of much interest until this period due to the
fact that all his needs were looked after. With encouragement
from his parents he starts to crawl, stand, and then walk.

A child is taught best when a game is made out of these learning habits to eliminate the frustration and boredom. He has a very short attention span and is therefore hard to teach. Patience is required by the parents, and the proper instructions as to the way a child should be encouraged to stand and walk is definitely a prerequisite for the parents. Remember, besides soft bones, the joints responsible for so much of the support and distribution of weight are still underdeveloped and cannot operate properly. When something is wrong at this early stage, it usually goes unnoticed because the child has no way of knowing something is wrong, and it is usually not visible to the parents. Later on in life, as he matures, so does the problem. It takes time for problems that stem from youth to be noticed, and then it takes time to correct them, if at all possible.

Proper feeding habits are also important throughout this stage to encourage growth. When a child does not receive proper nutrition, then this, too, plays a part in the poor working of the body. The body becomes starved for the right foods and tries to compensate in any way that is possible, and when it cannot, there is a malfunction that may show up in many ways. At this stage of the game, the five-year-old age bracket, the problems may already be too numerous to count. Structural and physiological damage may have already caused permanent damage either to internal organs or to the string and pulley system of muscles, ligaments, tendons, and cords that control the workings of our bodies.

The importance of growth is stressed in the six-to-teen years because the body shoots upward toward adult life, and changes take place that are sometimes too much for the child to cope with. The legs and arms become gangly and out of proportion, and the child becomes awkward in the control and balance of these parts.

This stage is a very active set of years when the youth is subjected to many knocks and bangs that may affect his growth. These bruises and sore muscles are superficially treated, and when the outward signs go away, we think the damage is fixed. However, silent damage — a shift in bone structure or a poor alignment of the skeletal frame due to a pulled ligament, cord, tendon, or muscle — may have occurred. Most of the time this damage is so slight that it goes unnoticed, becomes aggravated with adulthood, and this is what rolfers usually end up dealing with. The longer this type of damage exists, the more difficult it is to correct. It is the same as a broken bone that goes unattended for a period of time and then has to be rebroken to be corrected.

A small number of people have the incredible luck to go through life and reach retirement age without having the problems that the majority of us end up with, but they are very few and far between. If we would take the time out to learn about the human body and the causes and signs of a lot of structural problems, then we might be able to have the damage corrected before it becomes extreme, and we would end up feeling a lot better and living healthier lives.

Approaching middle age is like reaching a plateau in life. This group is more aware of their bodies because they have reached a stage where they are threatened with approaching old age and are afraid to acknowledge this fact. This is one of the most health conscious groups of people where health foods, jogging, and exercising in general have become very popular.

Mid-to-late fifties and on is a segment of life when not only the health of the body changes, but the mind along with it. People feel that they are coming to the end of the line. They have retired from work, edged out of many social functions, and do not have enough activity to fill their time. First of all, retirement is just moving into another stage of life, and if the right mental attitude is taken, there will probably be little change at all. "You are only as old as you feel." People let themselves stagnate and grow old long before their time. In order to replace the activity of work, you should have a hobby that could almost be turned into another career. If a hobby doesn't exist, there are many volunteer jobs that are always in need of extra help, and the age factor does not matter.

When approaching retirement, the first thing to do is to have a medical checkup and a re-evaluation. Proper care should be taken to re-establish good health in our bodies and minds.

Chapter 6

THE TECHNIQUES OF ROLFING

Rolfing is a technique that deals with all aspects of human behavior because any and all things affect us, either mentally or physically. One usually relates to the other in some way and to different degrees in each person. People are afraid to admit that they might have a problem and tend to compensate either by excuses or by hiding the problem and pretending there is nothing wrong. They even do it to the point where they become unaware that the problem exists any longer. The frustration of knowing that we are not performing as well as others makes us become self-conscious and hide within ourselves. The mind and the body deteriorate together unless constructive steps are taken.

Because rolfing takes a look at problems that affect both the physical and mental well-being, it is opening up a whole new medical approach. Remember, prevention should come first and foremost. It coincides with the way rolfers look at a patient in helping to distinguish the source of the problem. It relates to the person as a whole unit, as opposed to the way the medical profession treats only the damaged areas.

The art of rolfing or structural alignment of the body for good health was discovered by a woman named Ida P. Rolf. Medical science fixes or repairs the human structure when it breaks down, but it is only recently that science has begun to worry about the *causes* behind the breaking down and taking steps to *avoid* the breakdown. If a machine is running properly, there is less chance of its breaking down. Well, the same is true of the human body. If proper steps are taken to look after the body or corrective measures performed before damage results, then there is a probable chance that the human machine will not break down.

People feel that it is the organs of the body which keep us going. This is true to an extent, but it is the structural frame that holds and protects these vital organs. If this frame is in need of repair, it should be corrected before the organs it supports and protects are hurt. Our total mobility relies on our skeletal structure for without its smooth operation, our movement is restricted.

As the author of this book, I have done extensive research on the art of rolfing, including reading Ida P. Rolf's own book on the subject. I have talked to many people who have been rolfed and are rolfers themselves. My main concern with this new system of healing and making people feel better, generally, is the fact that it will make society sit up and take notice. With the high cost of living around the world today, more and more people are turning back to some of the old ways of sustenance which demand a more physical capability from each and every one of us. We are finding out that with new techniques coming along, we can *prevent* disorders in our systems that could not even be corrected properly in years past.

THE FEET

The feet present many problems from birth to death. They are constantly overworked and suffer great damage if not looked after. They support tremendous weight and pressure from above. The weight is focused on three main points in the form of a triangle. The peak or singular point is in the center of the heel while the other two are on either side of the foot at the base of the toes. The joint above the foot is the ankle; it is the working joint that supports the whole body weight and distributes the weight evenly out over the foot area. When the rolfer begins on the feet, he uses strong hand and finger manipulation to see that the bones are checked out and forced or snapped into place (Fig. 6-1).

THE ANKLE JOINT

The ankle is the main distributor of the weight so that it is spread evenly over the foot area to allow standing, walking, or running.

The feet support tremendous weight and pressure from above. Rolfing requires strong hand and finger manipulation to return the bones to their proper places and distribute the weight evenly on the three main points: the center of the heel and both sides of the feet at the base of the toes.

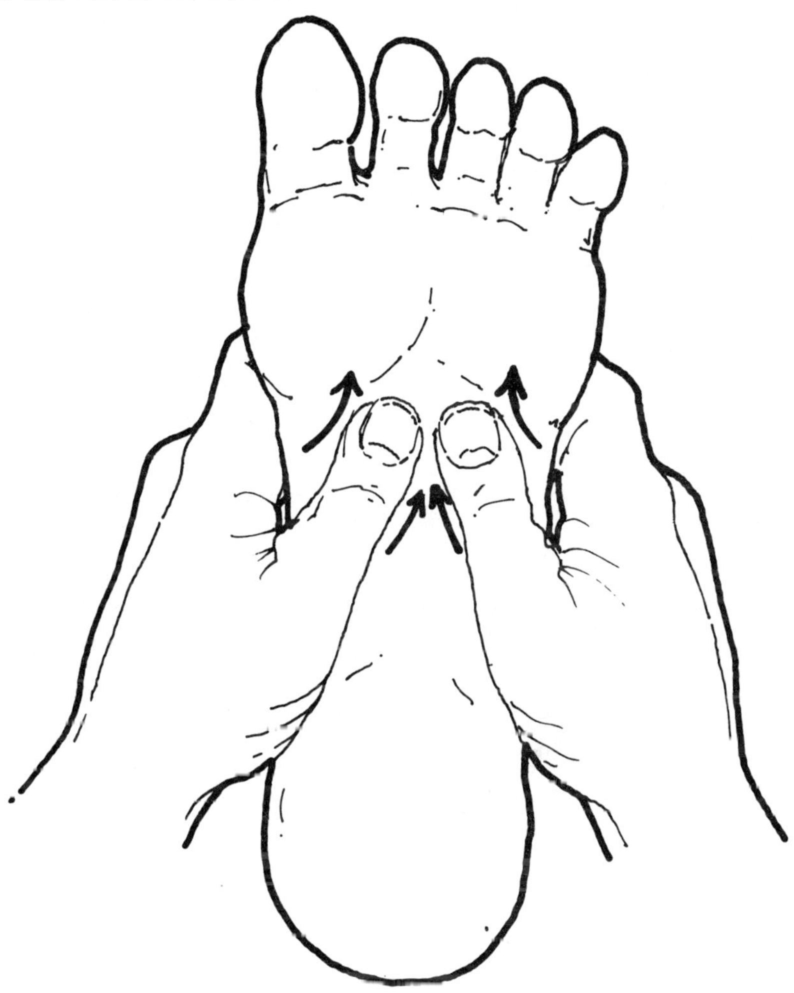

Figure 6-1

The leg is usually pulled lengthwise and cracked in order to separate the bones or even just to loosen them up. Then the muscles, tendons, ligaments, and cords are worked to make sure they are in good flexing order. The next step for the rolfer is to feel the bone structure with his fingers and to work the ankle joint at the same time to see if there is any grinding or misplacement of the joint. The base of the tibia, or lower part of the leg bone, must be centered over the ankle joint in order to support the weight of the body. Any disorder will either be pressed back into place by strong fingers or by the use of the palm of the hand (Fig. 6-2).

THE TIBIA AND FIBULA

The bones in the lower half of the leg are usually taken for granted unless one has been broken. This part of the leg has two main bones, the tibia and the fibula. The tibia is the larger of the two. It is at the front of the leg, joined at the knee on top and the ankle on bottom. This gives it a dual supporting job and makes it prone to being out of alignment. In a common fall, the ankle or the knee may twist, and due to the rigidity of the bone, it may easily be broken.

The lower part at the ankle is usually worked in conjunction with the rolfing of the ankle joint. Farther up at the knee joint, the leg must be checked for adhesions of muscle to the bone, and this is difficult in some people due to fatty buildup. The pressure of the fingers and hands involved in checking out this area may sometimes be painful, but it is necessary. The centered and connecting joints of the fibula (behind the tibia) must be checked and re-aligned if not in their proper positions in conjunction with the rest of the leg (Fig. 6-3).

THE KNEE

The knee is another connecting joint that is important in the balance and weight of the body. The knee is a kind of hinge that is

*The rolfer can feel the bone structure with his fingers,
work the ankle joint, and press any disorder
back into place. The ankle and leg are pulled
lengthwise and the muscles, tendons, and ligaments
worked to make sure they are in good flexing order.*

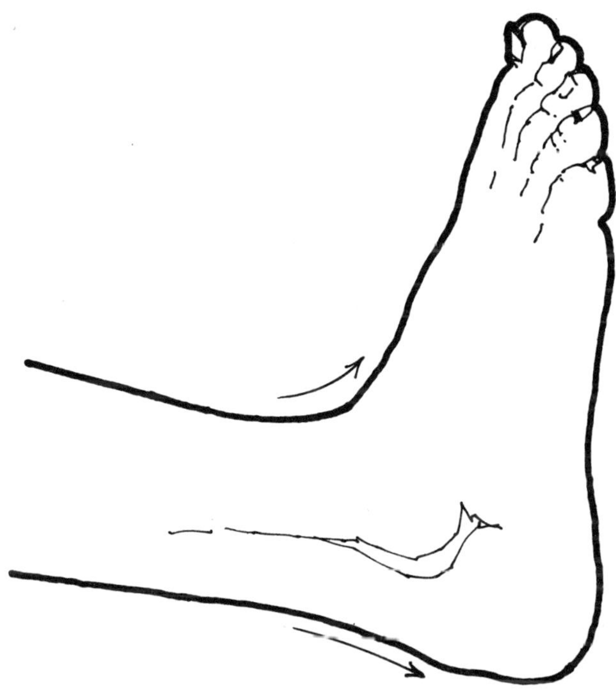

Pulling the ankle away
from the joint and
correcting the rotation

Figure 6-2

The bones in the lower part of the leg,
the tibia and fibula, are very prone to injury.
They are usually worked in conjunction
with the ankle joint. The pressure involved
in rolfing may be painful, but it is necessary.

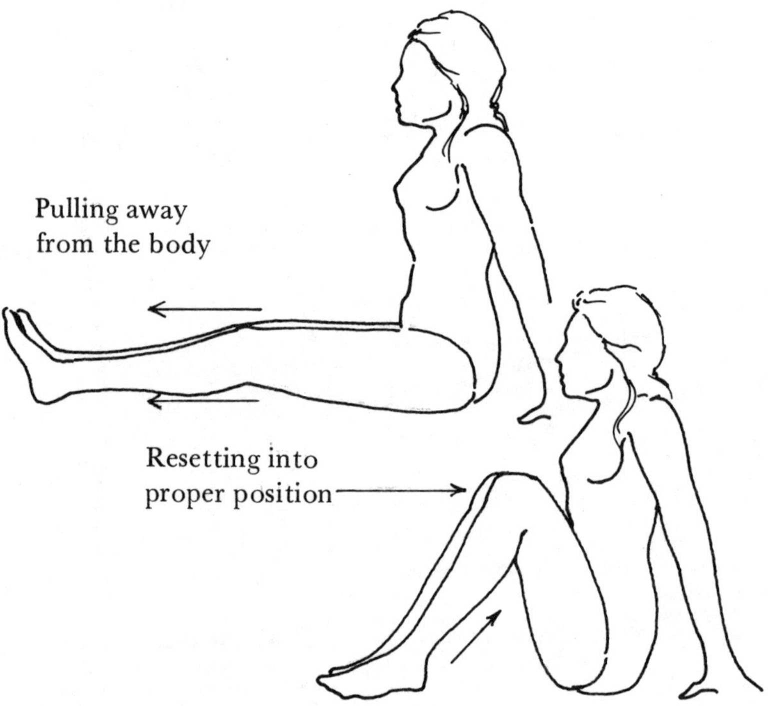

Figure 6-3

constructed for straight forward and backward movement. It is
the upper junction of the tibia, fibula, and femur or base of the
top half of the leg. The kneecap is simply a floating piece of cartilage known as the *patella*, and the whole knee joint, as we know
it, is encased in a mass of ligaments and tendons binding it together just as we would tape something in place. The palm of the hand
applying pressure, along with some vigorous pulling, is usually necessary for re-alignment (Fig. 6-4). If footprints are viewed, they
will, more than likely, reveal the knee joint's problem and the direction in which the rotation has occurred.

The knee joint, being so important in the lower structure, plays
a major part in the rotation or placement of the waist or pelvic
area. When the ankle joint is suffering from acute rotation, then
the foot itself will turn either inward or out to compensate for
this problem, but when the knee joint suffers from rotation, then
the waist or pelvic region usually works overtime to compensate
for the twist. If the knee joint is twisted outward, the waist is
pulled in the opposite direction in order to compensate for the outward pull of the knee joint. This condition also shows up in footprints (Fig. 6-5).

THE UPPER LEG AND HIP JOINT

When any of the previous problems exists in the lower part of the
leg, and rotation is seen in the pelvic region, the first part of the
skeletal structure that is affected is the hip joint or *femur* connection. This part of the upper bone is held in place with strong muscles and cords, and when rotation takes place, everything is twisted and pulled out of its proper place. Strain is exerted on all the
controlling factors — ligaments, muscles, cartilages, or cords. A
rolfer, in his corrective methods, may be forced to use his elbow
for extra strength or to exert his entire weight on this area in order to correct the positioning of the bone back into its central position in the socket (Fig. 6-6).

*The knee joint consists of a floating piece
of cartilage — the patella — and is encased in a mass
of ligaments and tendons. It is a kind of hinge
that not only allows movement in the legs,
but plays a major part in the rotation of the waist
or pelvic area. To rolf the knee, the palm of the hand
applies pressure along with some vigorous pulling.*

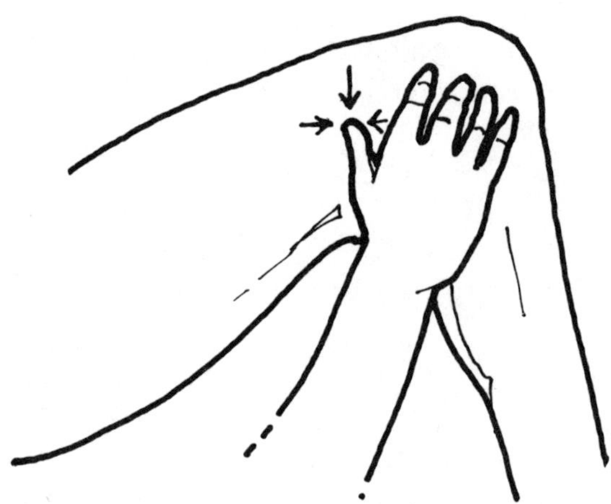

Figure 6-4

*Any rotation
in the ankle or knee
shows up in the
footprints.
The pelvis may
twist to
compensate for
the outward pull
of the knee joint,
and these twists
and pulls
are what show
in the feet.*

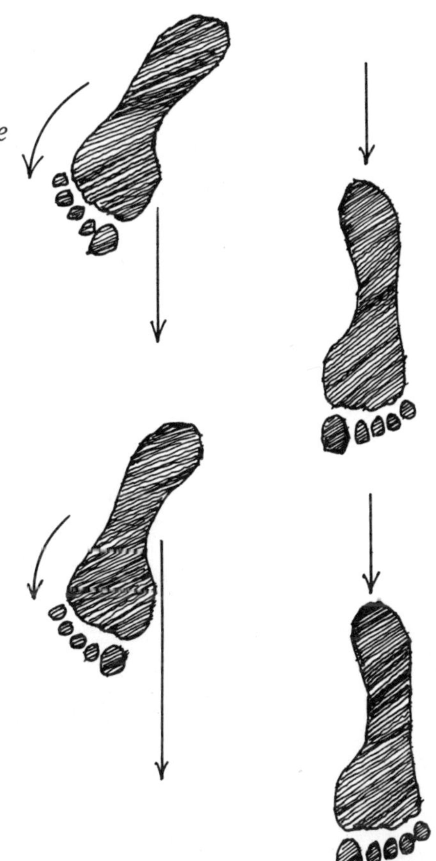

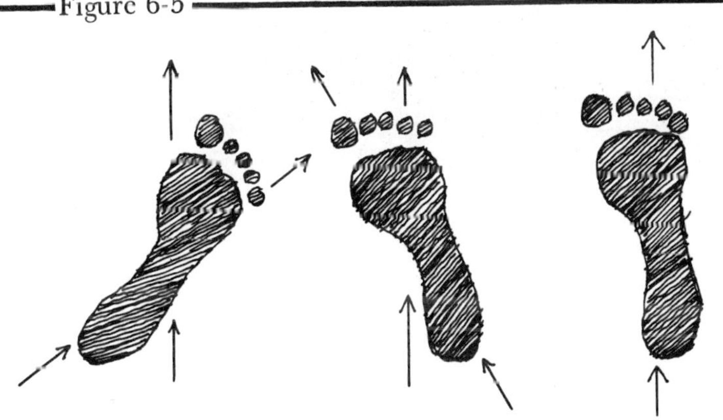

Figure 6-5

In correcting strain on the upper leg
and hip joint,
a rolfer must exert his entire weight
to re-align the bones,
ligaments, muscles, and cartilages.

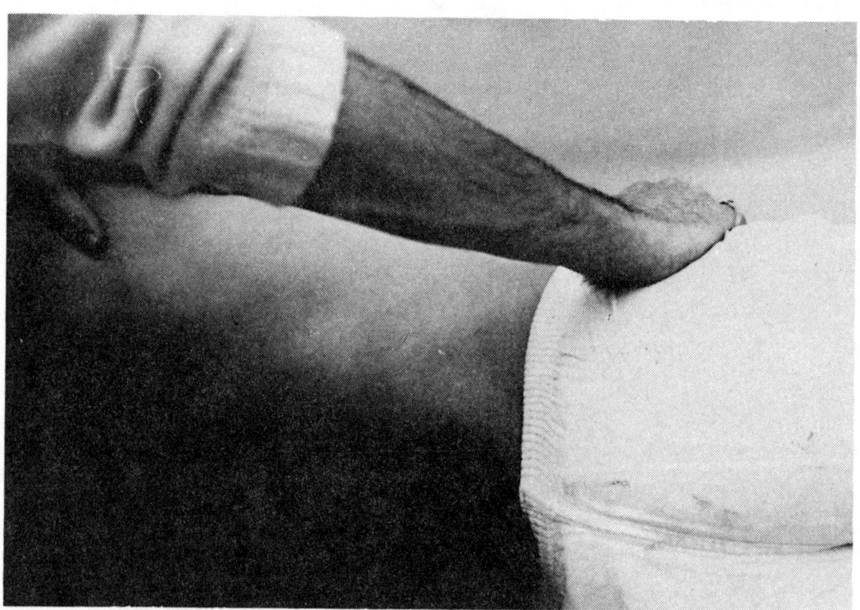

Figure 6-6

THE PELVIS

The pelvic region is referred to as the center of the whole structure because it balances and supports both the upper and the lower halves of the body. A lot of pressure is exerted on this area because it must support the total weight of the top half and evenly distribute it throughout the lower half. It is made up of many parts, and any one or several of these parts may be the cause of trouble. When one part is affected, no matter what the problem, then most likely it has had an effect on another section.

When the problem exists in the pelvic region, it is much more difficult to treat than in most other areas. A great deal of force must be exerted on some regions in order to re-align them into their proper positions. The rolfer may apply all of his force on the damaged area in order to slip the parts back into place or to release tension from jammed muscles or ligaments that have become distorted over a period of time. The elbow or the knee of the rolfer is an excellent source of strength to work with, providing proper care is taken to avoid damage from the extreme pressure (Fig. 6-7).

THE SPINE

The spine is the center of the whole upper part of the body and plays an important part in supporting the upper weight and the upright balance of the human structure. It travels from its pivoting lower connection to the pelvis, upwards in two arced curves, to a point under the center of the back base of the skull. Because of its central location, its main function, besides acting as a supporting beam for the upper half, is to take the top body weight and evenly distribute it throughout the lower half. The spine must maintain a central position and can be easily checked as to its ability to keep everything aligned just by looking and making sure that it is in line with the feet, pelvis, and the head. The vertebrae in the spine may be forced out of alignment with a light blow or

A problem in the pelvic region is difficult to treat.
A great deal of force must be exerted on the damaged area,
and the elbow or knee of the rolfer is an excellent source
of strength, but care must be taken
to avoid damage from the extreme pressure.

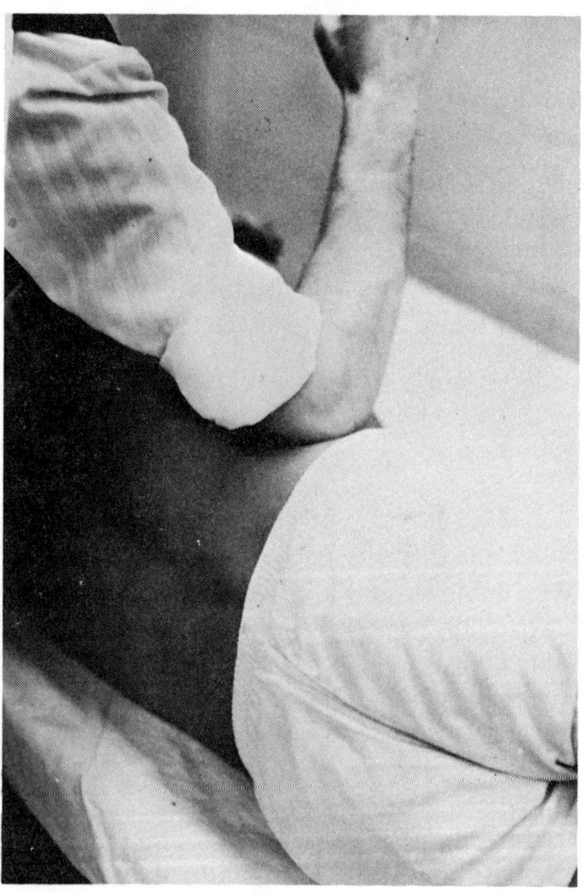

Figure 6-7

bump, and the nerve endings in the spine will then let us know by backaches or pain of some sort. It may even be felt in the feet. The vertebrae may be reset simply by forcing down with the palm on the offset vertebrae while the patient lies face down. Running the fingers together along the spine, while the individual is in this prone position and is relaxed, will usually locate the vertebrae which have moved (Fig. 6-8).

THE SHOULDER GIRDLE

In the shoulder area there are smaller bones which may be easily reset, if necessary, by using the fingers and the palm of the hand. The areas where the most damage occurs are the joints of the clavicles or collarbones and the direct shifting or dislocation of the humerus (upper arm bone) in the shoulder socket. Depending on the extent of the dislocation, the rolfer might be able to manipulate the area back into proper position or direct force may be used. One common way to rolf the shoulder is to sit on the floor with your legs straddling the patient, heels located one under the armpit and the other against the neck. This can be very dangerous if the rolfer does not know exactly what he is doing (Fig. 6-9).

THE CLAVICLE OR COLLARBONE

This is the protruding front bone that runs from the shoulder joint to the top of the sternum, just under the neck. There is one on each side of the chest. They are very weak, and it takes only about four to six pounds of hitting power to break or dislocate these bones. Forcing them back into place at the sternum area may result in severe chest pain. At the other end, a sore shoulder is the result, but immediate relief is felt (Fig. 6-10).

THE NECK

The neck area is an extension of the spinal column and is mostly affected by misplaced or altered vertebrae. Simple manipulation

*The rolfer runs his fingers along the spine
to locate any vertebrae which have moved.
They may be reset with the palm
while the patient lies face down and relaxed.*

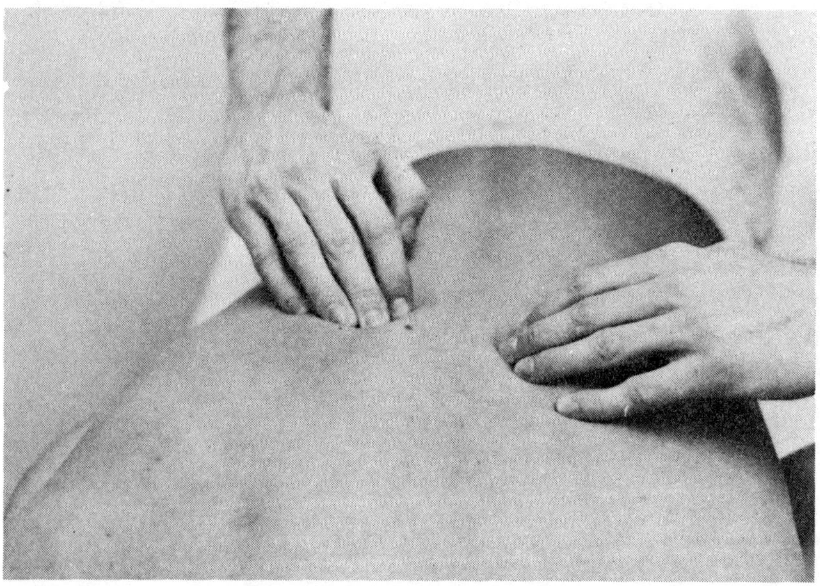

Figure 6-8

The shoulder sockets and collarbone

dislocate easily,

and the rolfer may be able to manipulate

the area back into position,

depending on the extent of the dislocation.

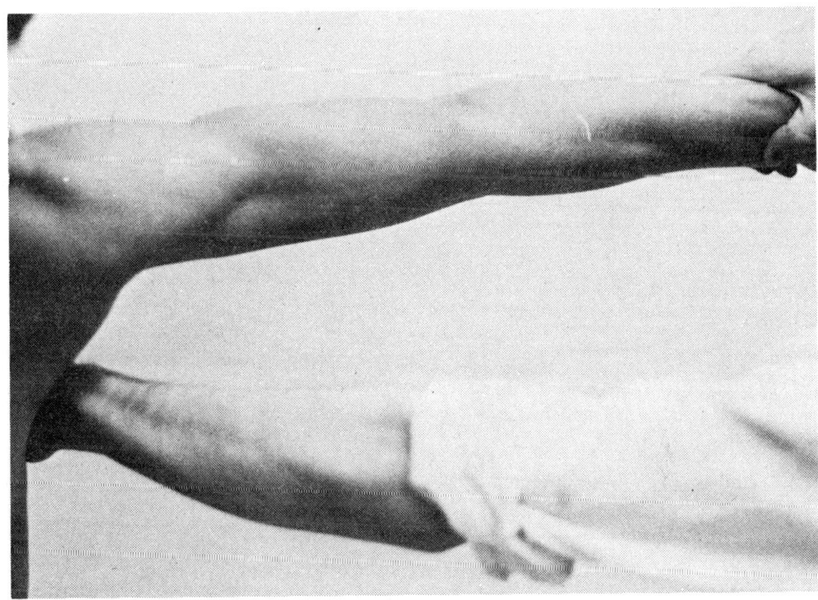

Figure 6-9

The collarbones or clavicles are very weak,
and it takes only about four to six pounds
of hitting power to dislocate these bones.
Severe chest pain may be the result of forcing them
back into place at the sternum, or a sore shoulder
may be the outcome at the other end,
but rolfing provides immediate relief.

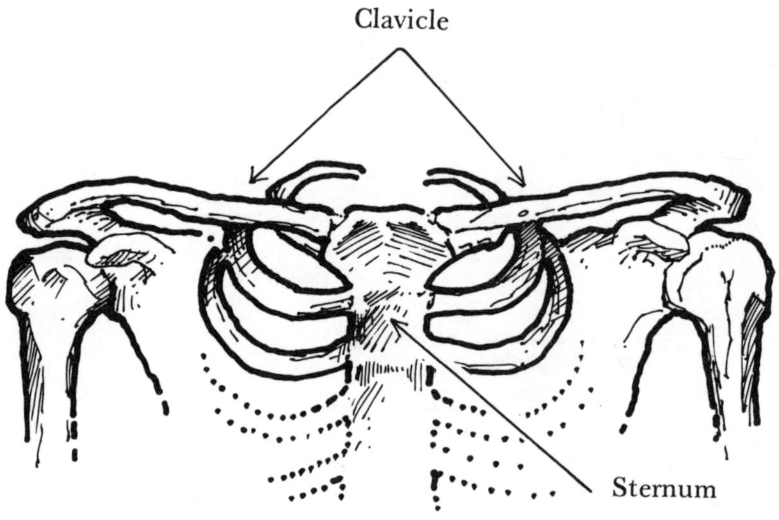

Figure 6-10

*Extreme caution must be used in rolfing
the vertebrae of the neck. These vertebrae
are an extension of the spinal cord,
and although simple manipulation, along with
a violent jerk of the neck, usually brings relief,
no beginner should attempt this maneuver.*

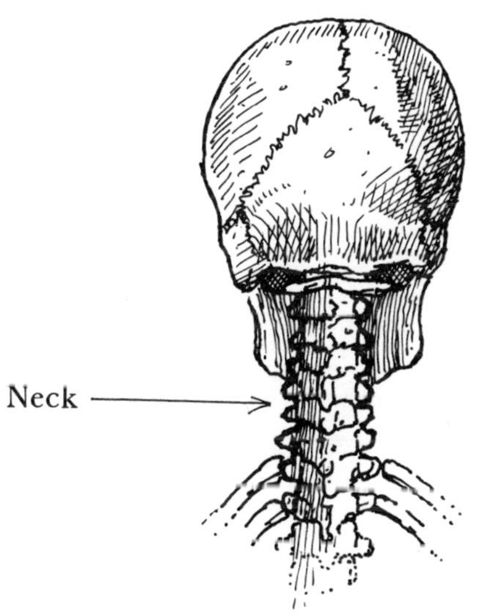

Figure 6-11

of these vertebrae with the hands, along with a violent jerk of the neck, usually resets any out-of-place vertebrae, and immediate relief is felt. Extreme caution should be exercised, and *no* beginner should attempt this manipulation (Fig. 6-11).

In summing up, I would just like to say that I have tried to give you, the reader, a rough idea as to how the treatment of rolfing may be applied. Not all cases are the same. Different people have different medical problems accompanying their disorders.

Basically, it all concerns our mobility. Without each part of the body operating efficiently, movement is impossible. If one leg is damaged, the other one works twice as hard to compensate. The same is true of the arms. Inside the body, the muscles, cartilages, cords, and tendons do the same.

Chapter 7

COMMENTARY ON STRUCTURALLY ALIGNING THE BODY

Since rolfing deals with setting the human structure back into better balance with the earth's gravitational downward pull in order for it to perform more effectively, then after the body has been aligned the result is usually a better and lighter feeling throughout. This lighter sensation is the first step toward better health. From there on begins a psychological change that makes for further improvement. Rolfing itself can be a very painful process because it takes great force or pressure to create the changes necessary, and the many people who have been rolfed, or the rolfers themselves, attest to this fact. Even though they have been through pain, they still promote rolfing as something that is very good for everyone.

Most people, short of those born with actual physical defects, have a pattern in which they develop and grow, both physically and psychologically. Development may continue, or deterioration may set in. Remember that the body is a bag of bones, sinew, and liquid, encased in an envelope of skin. If it is not operating as a whole unit, it has to work harder, and more vital energy is used. Other parts have to work overtime to compensate. This leads to deterioration of the part that is compensating for the damaged area, or cessation of function altogether.

All operating parts of the human structure must be situated in their respective places in order to achieve the potential that the body is built for. This procedure begins from the ground up like the construction of a house. If there is a weak foundation, the unit may collapse. When the construction is completed, there is a tremendous downward force on the base due to the gravitational pull of the earth. This is true in our bodies as well. The downward gravitational pull is constant. When a segment of skeletal structure is out of alignment, it is pulled down by gravity so it misses the point it is supposed to rest upon, and a problem becomes evident. This, in turn, affects the emotional state of the individual.

In rolfing, the rolfer begins at the foundation of the construction, the base, and works upward, re-aligning the pieces in order to set every part back into proper working order. As the pieces are properly reconstructed in their rightful places, the psychological mood of the individual is transformed. In rolfing, we are dealing with the human being as a whole, not just in part, as the physician does. When you reflect inwardly and something is wrong, it shows outwardly, simply by the way you carry yourself.

An unhappy person may not have a medical problem, but when a medical problem exists, even though he is unaware of it, then the character, mood, or personality of the individual changes. A simple example is someone with a toothache or a headache. This individual is certainly not the most pleasant company. The minute his problems are corrected, his whole mood undergoes a change. This is basically the same in rolfing. When someone is rolfed, he immediately feels better and behaves accordingly.

It has been said that man is the only animal who adjusts to his surroundings. This may be true, but he then adjusts to his own defects as well. Constructively the defects must be readjusted to fit the man in order for the man to operate as he was intended. When a man changes physically, he changes psychologically as well, and when he is readjusted physically, his psychological outlook must be readjusted.

The growth pattern is set at birth. If it is changed, growth does not stop, but the individual continues to develop incorrectly. If he is rolfed back into proper health, then he will continue in that proper way, unless something else is induced to change the pattern again. Rolfing is not necessarily permanent.

The following illustration shows a defect in the vertebrae (Fig. 7-1). We sometimes take this for granted. In structural re-alignment through the technique of rolfing, the whole framework must

A defect in the vertebrae may be taken for granted.
Even the resultant backaches and headaches
may be adjusted to, but a physical change causes
a psychological change as well. Rolfing the spine
back into alignment, therefore, improves
the patient's psychological outlook, too.

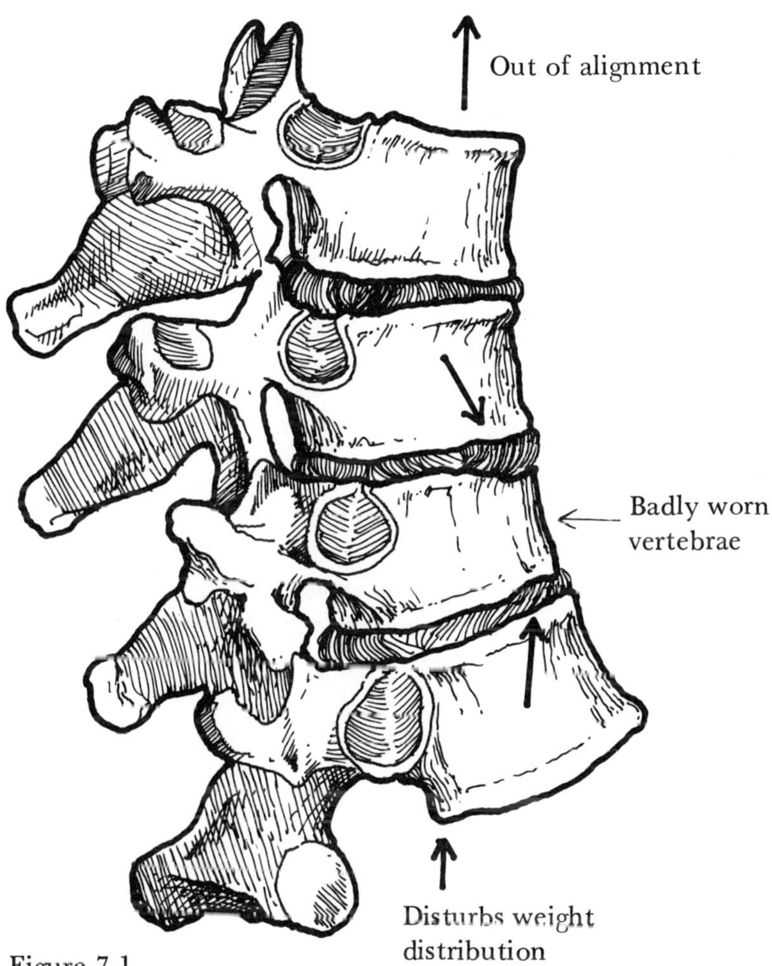

Figure 7-1

be done in order to balance and tune its respective parts.

By looking at footprints or at the feet themselves, the story of the individual may be told, in that any problems existing in the upper structure usually end up showing in the lower structure. Telltale signs appear in the footprints. Everything may be read in the feet (Fig. 7-2).

Strain and improper balance may also be seen in the legs of the individual. The foot itself is affected by the rotating process that may exist in the waist or the knee joints. The rotation may be inward or outward and take place at either spot or in both. The individual simply states that this is the way he walks and will consider it normal (Fig. 7-3). In the meantime, strain has been placed on other areas to help compensate for the loss suffered in the shift of the person's downward weight pull.

The weight and the back pull of the muscles in someone who is not structurally balanced affects his ability to bend in various directions. Most of us are under the erroneous impression that an overweight person cannot bend or flex as easily as others. This is not usually the case except in extreme obesity. The problem lies within the structure of the back and the flexibility of the tendons, cords, and muscles involved in the bending and flexing process. Structural alignment corrects these problems, and total freedom in the waist and back is usually felt for the first time (Fig. 7-4).

When someone is in the process of bending forward, the muscles in the stomach area should be flexing to the point where they are shortening and forming a fatty, drooping extension in a downward direction of the stomach. This means that they are performing properly. In an athlete, the muscles may simply tighten rather than droop due to the hardening process they have been subjected to. The back should be pulled flat as the muscles are stretched lengthwise. If a board is placed on the back of someone who is bent over, there should be no spaces through which light may shine. The board should lie perfectly flat. When examining an individual in this position, notice that the muscles in the backs of the legs, behind the kneecaps, are outstretched, trying to give the

*Strain on the feet is the result
of damage anywhere in the body,
and the rolfer always examines
the footprints for telltale signs.*

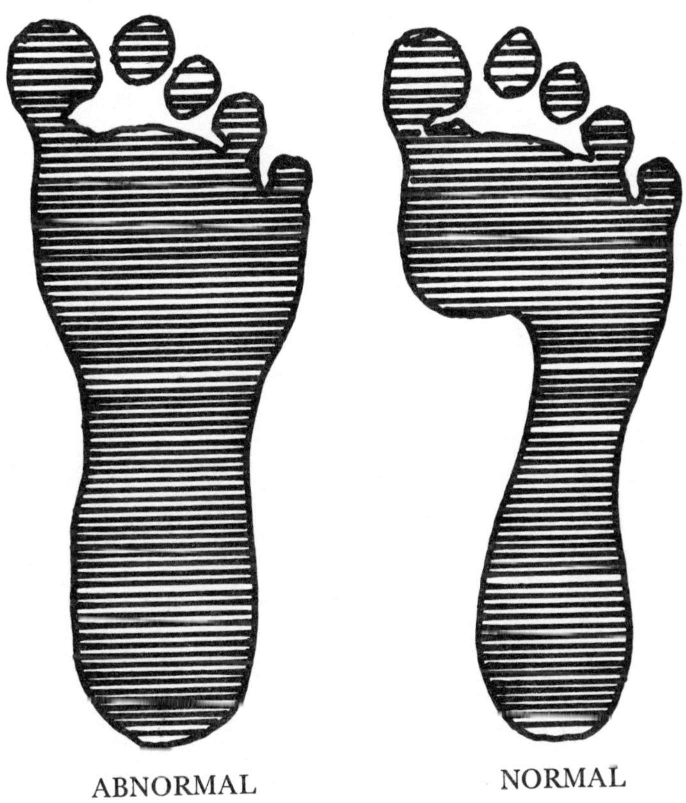

Figure 7-2

*The legs also show the consequences
of strain and improper balance.
An uncomfortable gait
is usually merely taken for granted.*

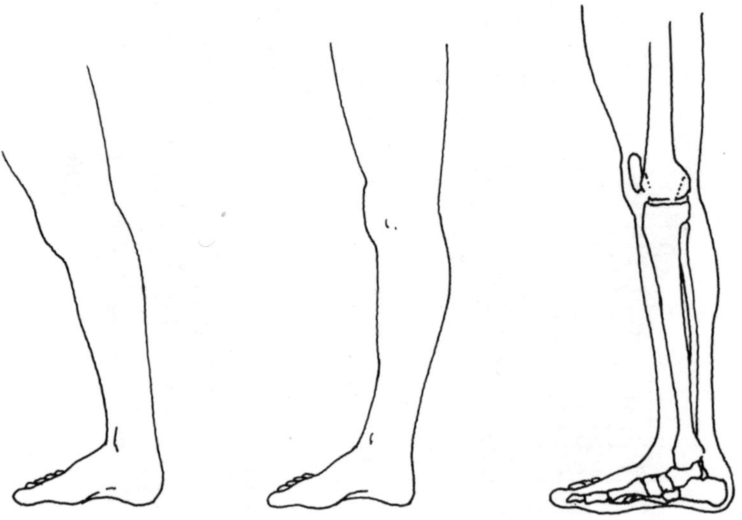

Figure 7-3

Structural alignment of the back
makes bending and flexing much easier.
The waist and back area should feel
totally free and relaxed. When the muscles
behind the knees tighten,
limited bending is the result.

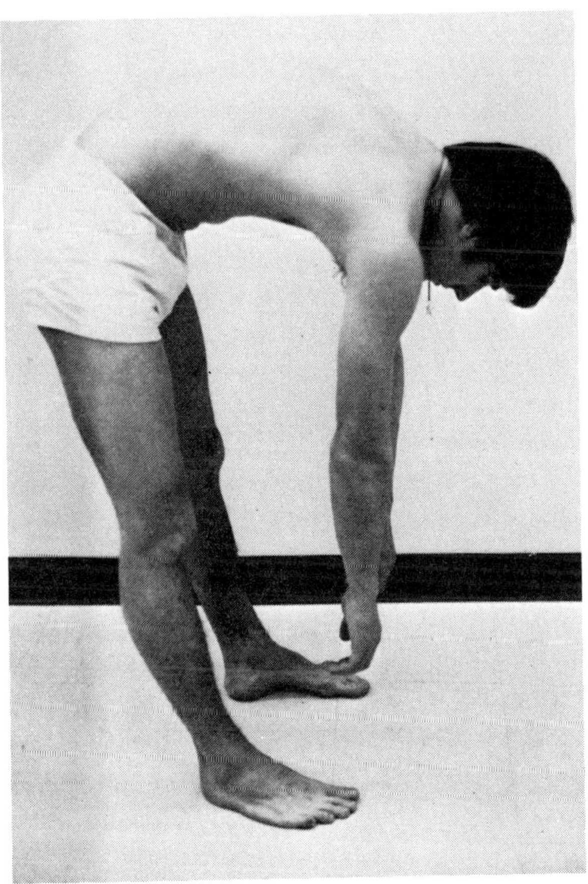

Figure 7-4

body the flexibility it needs in order to bend over. If these muscles do not possess the ability to stretch in conjunction with the rest of the structure, then limited bending is the result. This lack of ability to bend over properly shows that the muscles have not been exercised properly and lack the flexibility they should have.

The same may be said of bending backward with the exception that due to the skeletal structure and the lack of joints in the back of the body, the ability to bend backward is limited. If our joints had the ability to bend as much in both directions, we would be able to double ourselves over backward.

Breathing properly is important when exercises are performed. When we hold our breath while performing an exercise, we expand the lungs and restrict the ability of the joints to "give" properly to the bend. If air is inhaled first and slowly exhaled as the exercise is performed, then there are no restrictions on the joints.

The following illustrations demonstrate the problems involved in bending forward and backward. Note where the restrictions exist (Figs. 7-5 and 7-6). Also note the arc in the curve of the body in the backward bend and the actual doubling in half of the individual in the forward bend. All muscles controlling the bending ability are flexing and stretching muscles, and there are no restrictions from the joints.

Due to poor posture or through accident or disease, curvatures of the spine, horizontal or vertical, slight or extreme, appear in many individuals. Tilting of the head due to misplacement of the pelvic area may cause the spinal column to give in to the downward pressure and force the spinal vertebrae to become distorted. When this condition exists, no matter how slight, steps must be taken to correct it immediately, or else it will have some effect on the rest of the structure. If it appears in a child due to disease or accident, then the child should be allowed to reach adulthood before any necessary surgery is performed. Rolfing sometimes straightens the malformation in the child without surgery.

The rolfing process may be painful, but when the patient is a child, and the body is still soft and the bones flexible, then it is corrected with less difficulty. If the patient is an adult, then the

The ability to bend backward is limited.
Note the arc in the curve of the body.
All muscles controlling bending ability
are flexing and stretching.

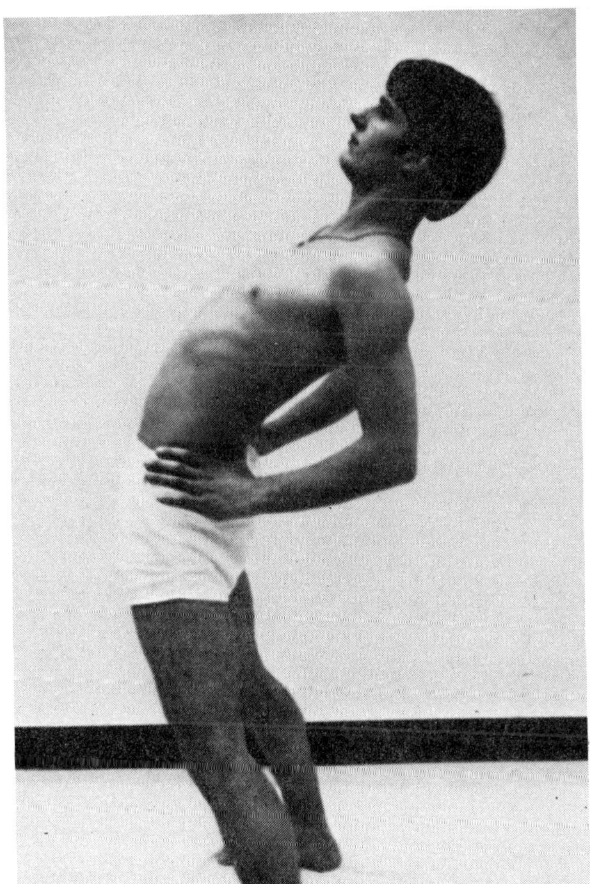

Figure 7-5

*During exercising, proper breathing
is important. If air is inhaled first and
slowly exhaled as the exercise is performed,
then there are no restrictions on the joints.*

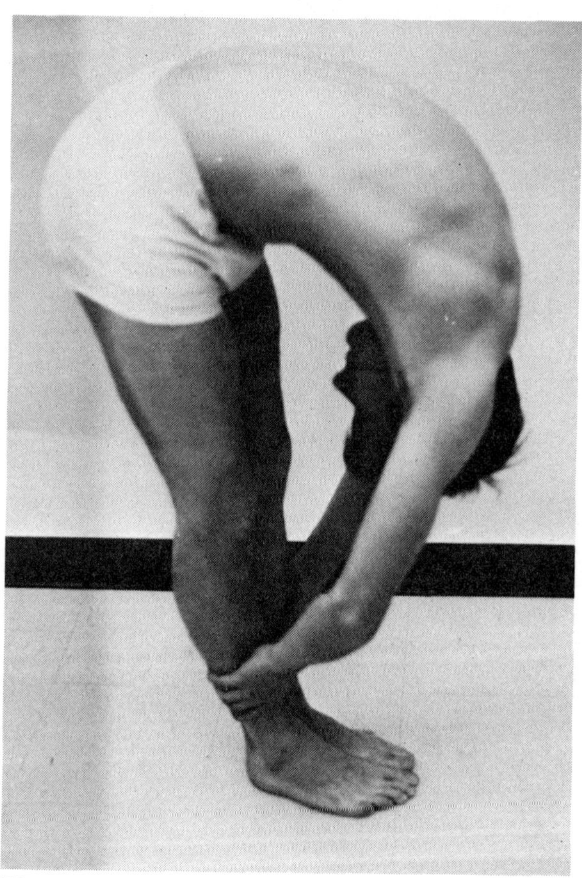

Figure 7-6

growth process has stopped, and the curvature has had a longer time in which to settle. It is then more difficult. More than likely, other sections of the structure have also been affected due to the misplacement of weight over the entire body.

After treatment in the spine and pelvic region has been performed over a period of time, the pieces are aligned, and the body has the ability to stand erect once more (Figs. 7-7 and 7-8).

The muscles are affected when the spine and the pelvic region are in trouble, throwing the head off center on its axis above the body. The neck usually takes on a craned look and exerts its downward force in front of the body pulling the top half of the torso forward. A forward tilt of the pelvic area can cause the shifting of the rib cage and the relaxing of the sterno-cleido-mastoid muscle leading into the neck from the top of the rib cage to the back of the base of the skull (Fig. 7-9).

Reconstruction from the feet up must take place in order for every part to be placed back into balance. Then the head will slowly begin to settle back over its proper center. The following drawings show before and after effects of a short period of rolfing treatments (Figs. 7-10, 7-11, 7-12, and 7-13).

Not everyone is in need of rolfing, even though the signs of a problem may exist. Remember that there are people who feel they have a problem only after they have been told of the symptoms. Medical students suffer a great deal from this psychological effect during their training in medicine. The more they find out about various illnesses, the more they are sure they have them.

Many people are being trained in rolfing, and it is only a matter of time before one will be within your home area. Before anyone is subjected to rolfing, he is given an evaluation examination so the rolfer has a general idea as to which area needs the most concentration. This is just like any medical examination.

Rolfing is similar to chiropractic except that the chiropractor usually treats only the afflicted area. This leaves the rest of the body structurally out of balance with the corrected area. Rolfers start at the bottom and work up through the damaged area making sure there is a balance throughout the whole body. The

Curvatures of the spine — horizontal or vertical,
slight or extreme — appear in many individuals.
They are due to poor posture, accident, or disease.
The rolfing process may be painful, but treatment
will enable the body to stand erect once more.

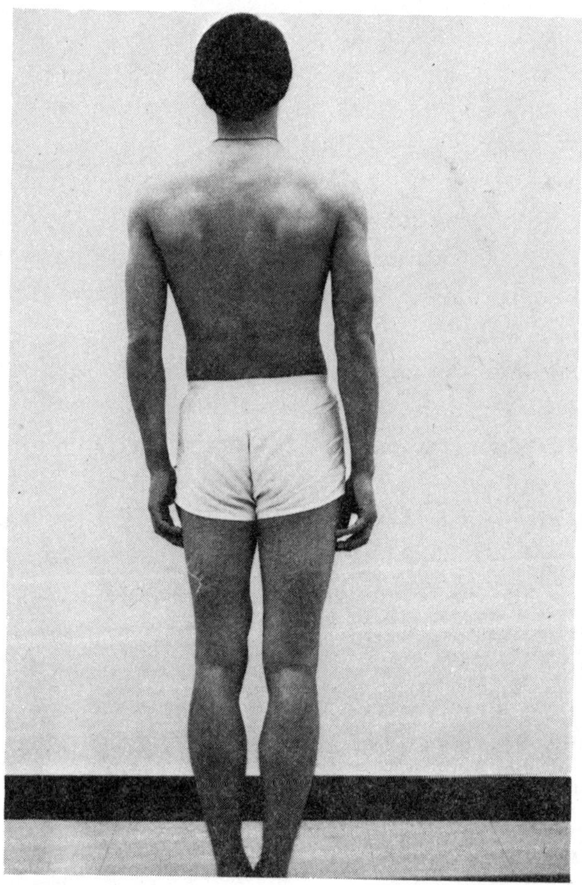

Figure 7-7

In an adult, a curvature of the spine has had
a long period of time in which to settle.
This makes the rolfing treatment more difficult
and may take a long period of time to correct.

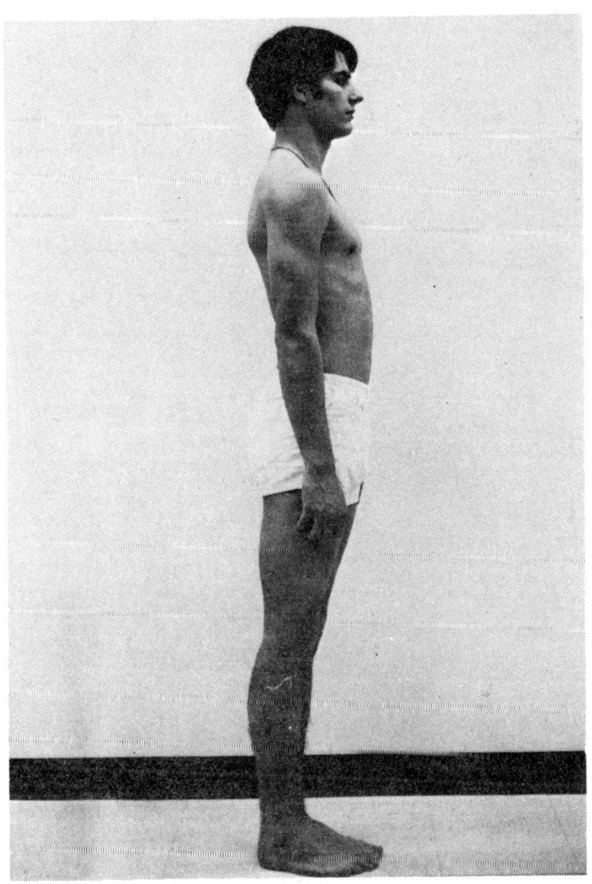

Figure 7-8

*A forward tilt of the pelvic area can cause a shifting
all the way up to the sterno-cleido-mastoid muscle
leading into the neck from the top of the rib cage
to the back of the base of the skull. The head and
neck pull forward, causing a stoop and a craned look.*

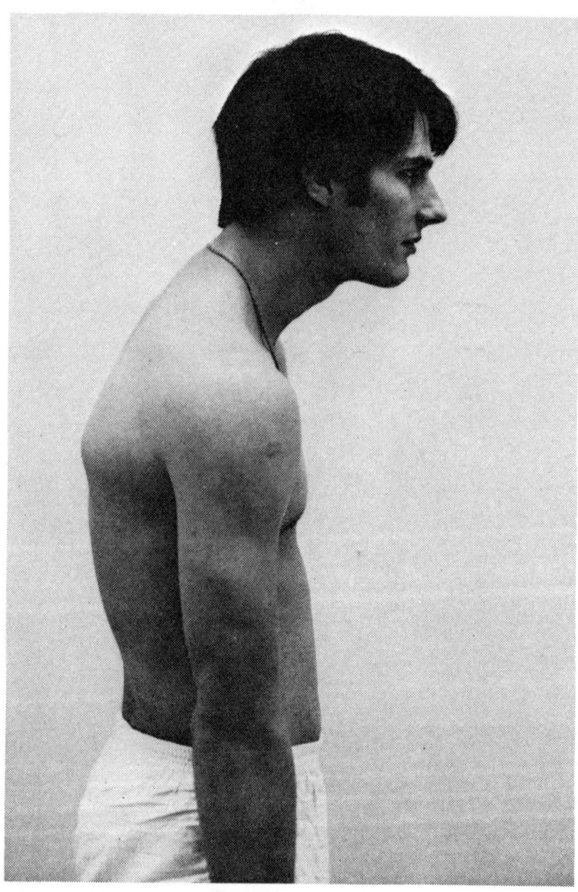

Figure 7-9

*After a short period of rolfing treatments,
there is already an improvement.
The head and shoulders are more erect,
and the spine is straighter.*

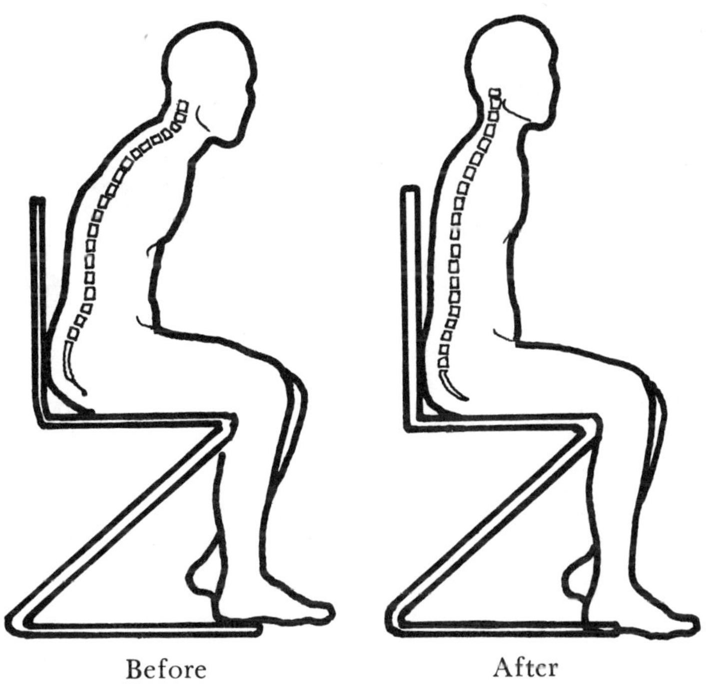

Figure 7-10   SITTING

When the shoulders are in a straight line,
the muscles of the back are relaxed.
The aches and pains that accompany
a "bad back" disappear. Sometimes these pains
are blamed on arthritis, bursitis, or rheumatism,
but are actually the result
of a spine that is out of alignment.

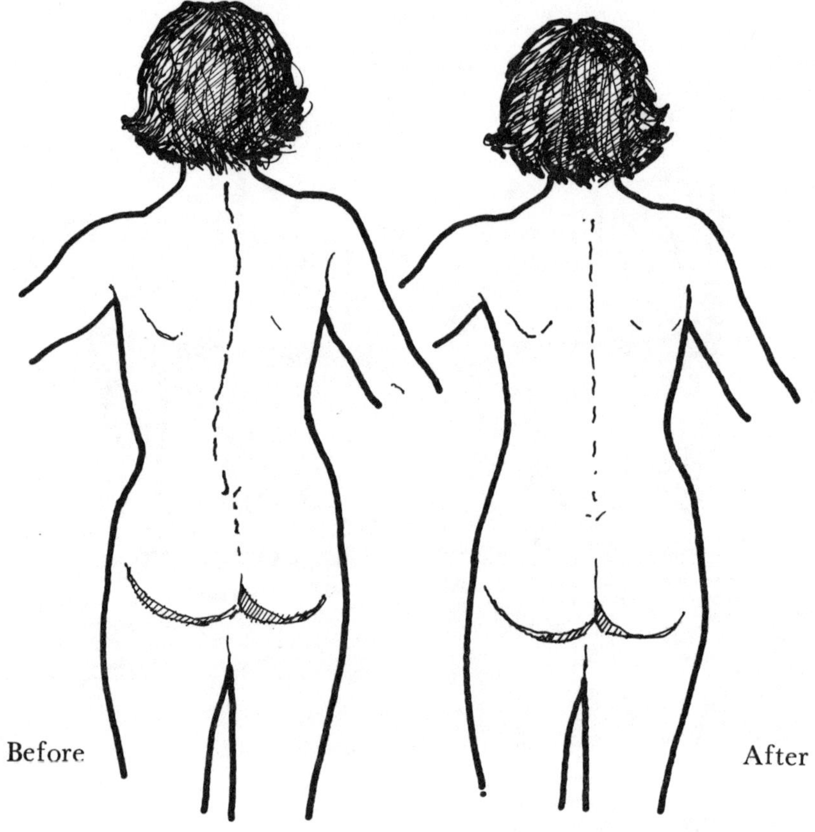

Before   After

Figure 7-11   STANDING

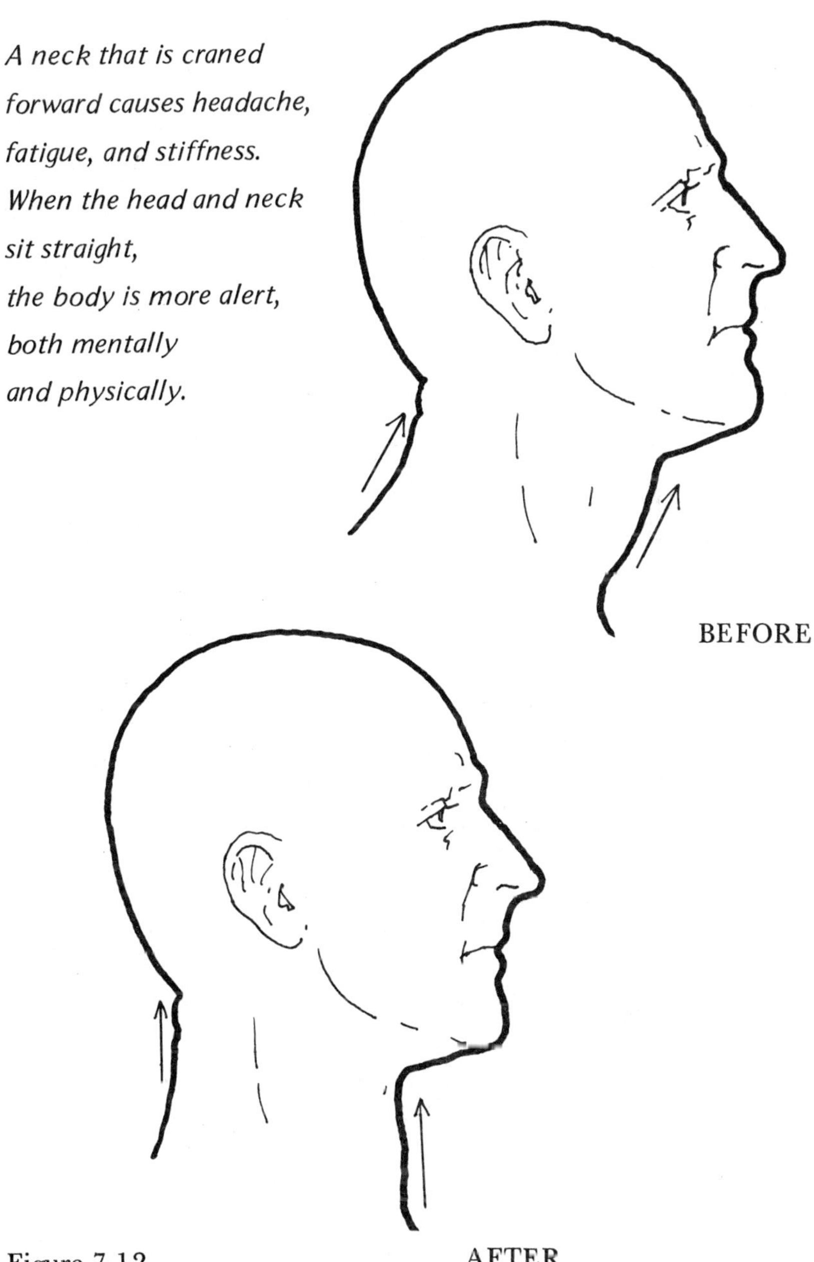

*A neck that is craned
forward causes headache,
fatigue, and stiffness.
When the head and neck
sit straight,
the body is more alert,
both mentally
and physically.*

Figure 7-12

The body looks better when the abdomen is flat and the back is straight. Even without weight loss, it also looks more slender. Looking and feeling better creates a healthier outlook.

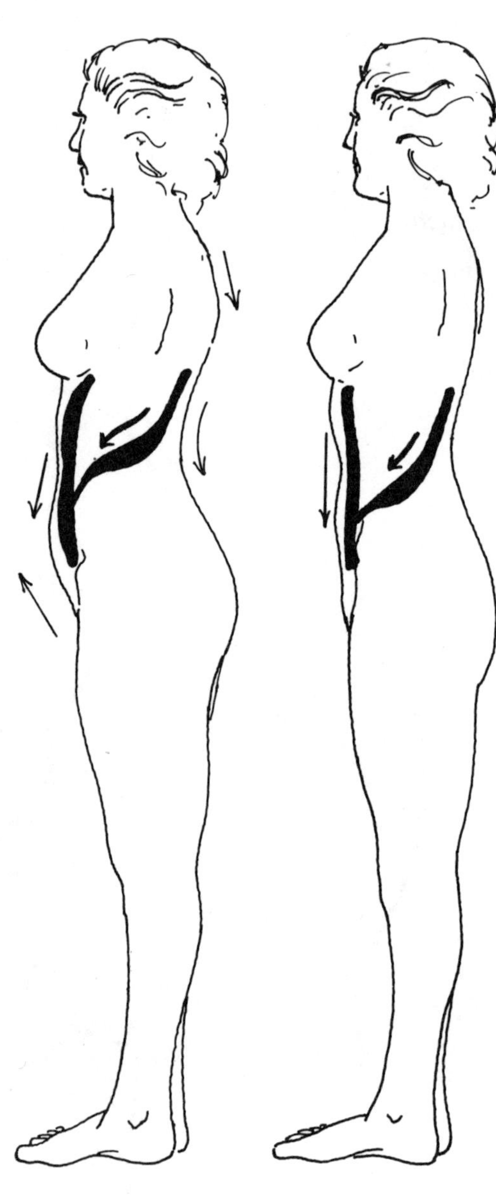

Figure 7-13

illustrations show proper alignment while the body is in motion (Figs. 7-14, 7-15, 7-16, and 7-17).

A rolfing session takes about ten hours, depending on the condition of the body. It is much easier to rolf a body that is in pretty good shape as opposed to one that is obese and has many problems.

Most individuals feel wonderful after they have been rolfed. They possess better balance and are more relaxed psychologically. The result is a changed person with an improved outlook on life.

Rolfing starts at the bottom and works all the way up through the entire body, not just the afflicted area. Whether the part is in motion or at rest, it must be structurally aligned. Good health is the result of the entire structure functioning as one unit.

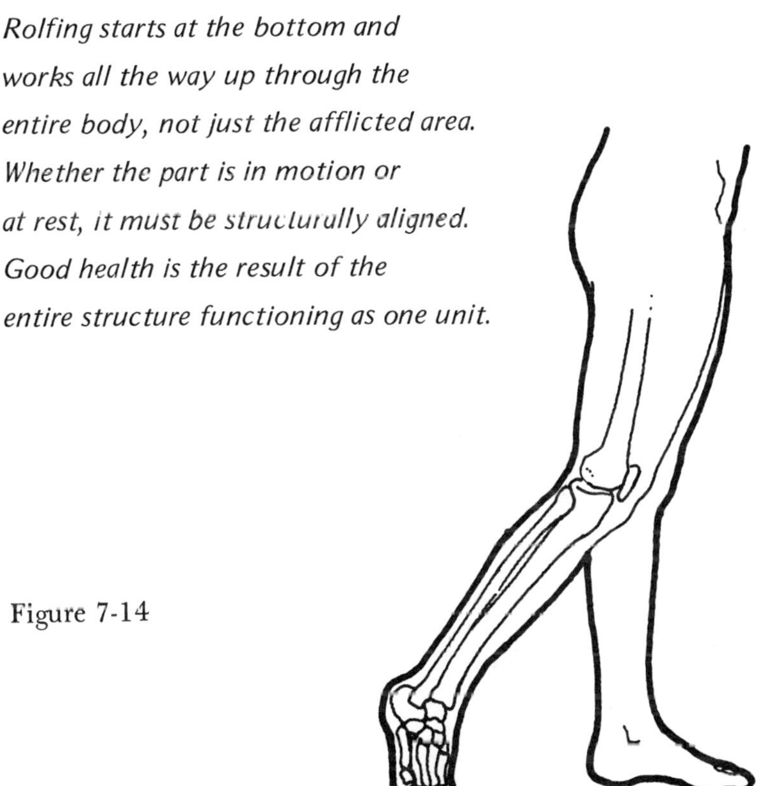

Figure 7-14

ANKLE MOVEMENT

From the feet up through the pelvis, these bones
are all aligned and able to withstand the weight of the
entire body. Restricted movement in one part
of the body always affects another area.
The constant strain and shifting in the healthy areas,
trying to compensate for the damaged ones,
results in further damage.

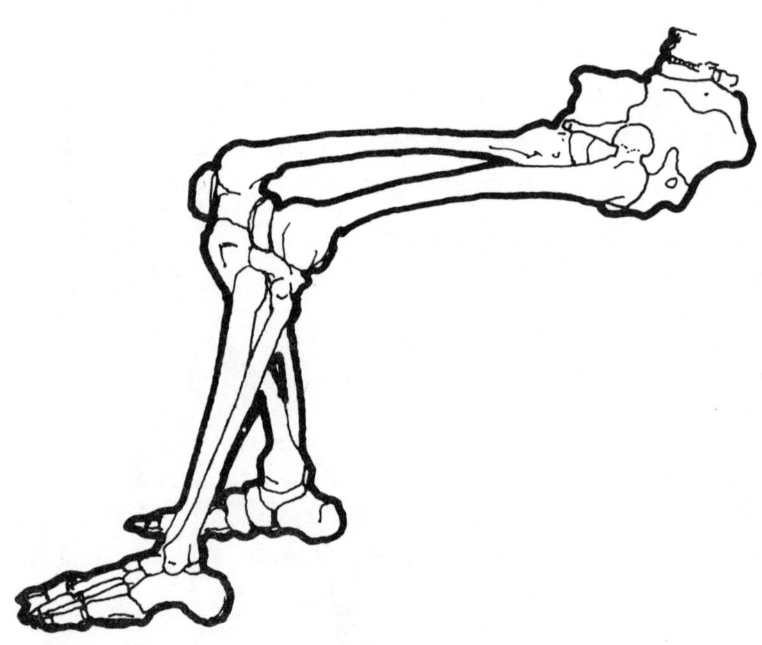

Figure 7-15   KNEE MOVEMENT

*The pelvis is the center of balance, receiving pressure
from above and distributing it evenly below.
A problem that appears in one area may actually be
coming from another one. A rolfer gives
an evaluation examination to determine
what area of the body needs the most work.*

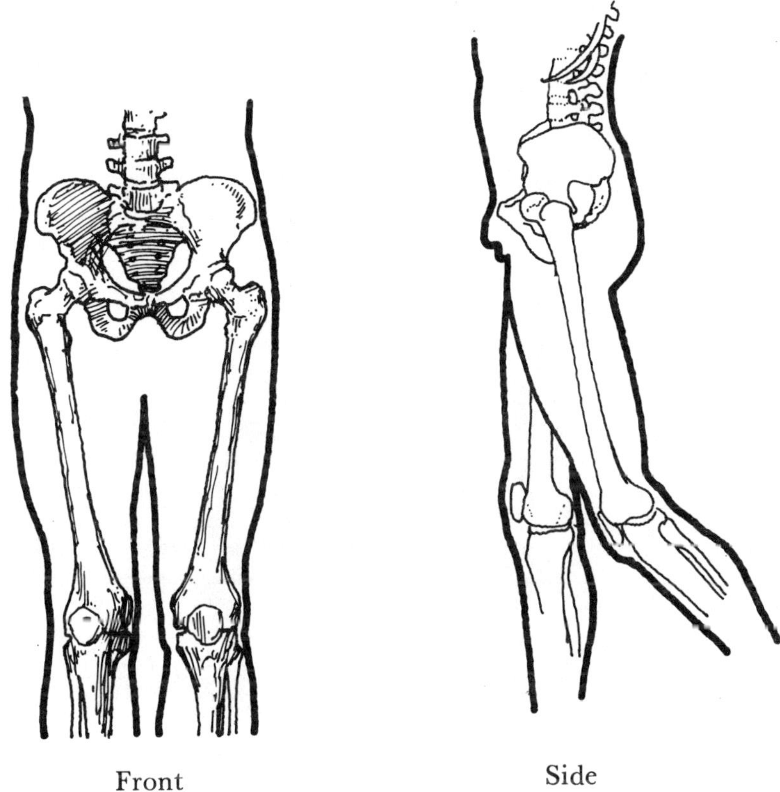

Front   Side

Figure 7-16   PELVIC MOVEMENT

Many problems occur in the spinal column,
but the rolfer treats the entire body.
A rolfing session takes about ten hours,
depending on the condition of the body.

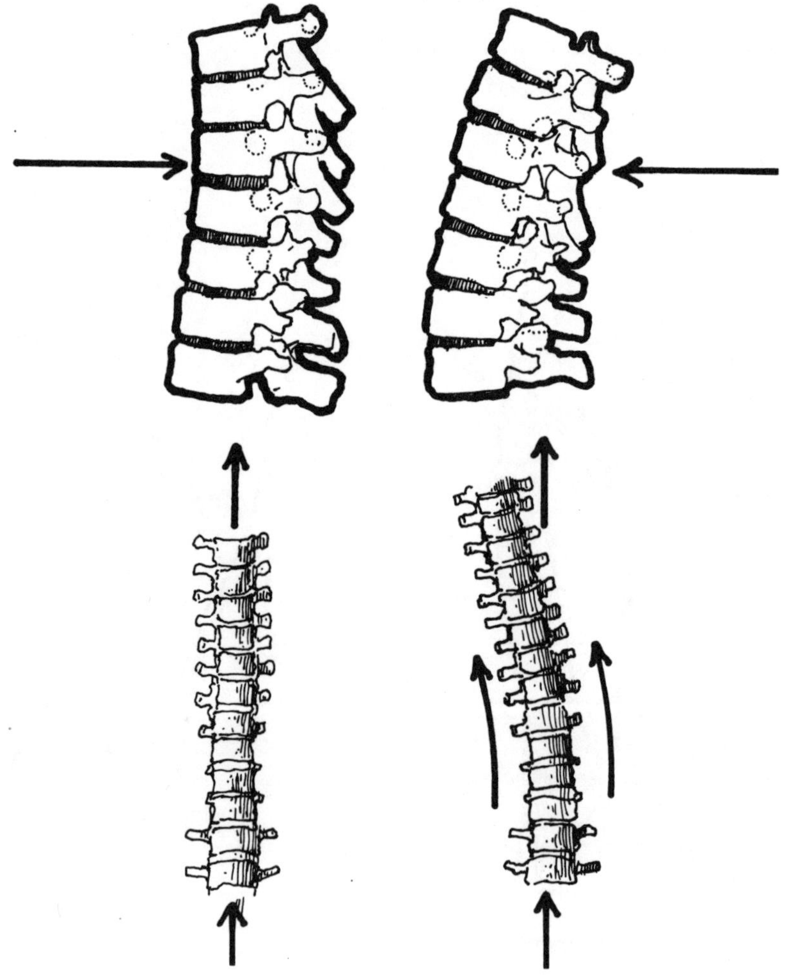

Figure 7-17   SPINAL MOVEMENT

index